A Guide to Hormonal Dermatology

Ramanjit Singh • Nidhi Sharma
Editors

A Guide to Hormonal Dermatology

Foreword by
Torello Lotti
Naresh Trehan

Springer

Editors
Ramanjit Singh
Senior Consultant
Medanta Hospital
Gurgaon, India

Nidhi Sharma
Senior Consultant Dermatologist
Skin Health Clinic
Gurugram, Haryana, India

ISBN 978-981-99-7717-8 ISBN 978-981-99-7715-4 (eBook)
https://doi.org/10.1007/978-981-99-7715-4

This Springer imprint is published by the registered company Springer Nature Singapore Pte Ltd.
The registered company address is: 152 Beach Road, #21-01/04 Gateway East, Singapore 189721, Singapore

Dedicated to my loving family and friends for their unconditional love and support

And a Special Thanks to the Editor Dr Ramanjit Singh for his faith and wise guidance at each and every step of this project.

I express my appreciation to the authors of the chapters for their submissions and interest in this publication.

A sincere thanks to My Patients who have shown trust in me and given me an opportunity to treat them and become a capable doctor.

Last but not least, I thank Springer Publication House especially Ms Raman, Mr Naren, and Ms Suganya for their unfailing cooperation and courtesy.

Foreword 1

Dermatology's realm extends far beyond skin-deep, as the profound influence of hormones on skin health and appearance comes to light. This dynamic interplay forms the cornerstone of the intricate relationship between dermatology and hormones. The intricate relationship between skin and hormones is a captivating tale of biology's influence on our appearance and identity.

As scientific understanding evolves, innovative hormone-based treatments emerge, redefining possibilities in skincare. This synergy between dermatology and hormones is a captivating journey, unravelling the delicate balance between our body's internal regulatory systems and the external reflections seen in our skin. A deeper exploration of this liaison promises insights that transcend traditional beauty, offering a holistic understanding of human health and vitality.

This book is organized to provide a comprehensive overview of our understanding of the mechanism of hormones in dermatology. It is hoped that this book will fill the void that currently exists in the understanding of various hormone-related diseases, especially polycystic ovarian syndrome (PCOS), diabetes, and skin, thyroid disease and skin, obesity and skin, providing a better understanding for the management of these conditions.

I acknowledge the work of Dr Ramanjit Singh and Dr Nidhi Sharma, and we are very grateful for the energy and hard work that they put into making this book come into existence.

We hope that you enjoy reading this book, and the knowledge gained from this work may provide an impetus for future discovery in hormonal treatment and lead to improvements in the care of our patients with various skin diseases.

Rome, Italy — Torello Lotti

Foreword 2

I give my heartfelt thanks to the Editors Dr Ramanjit Singh and Dr Nidhi Sharma and all other contributing authors for giving me the opportunity to write the foreword to this excellent book on *A Guide to Hormonal Dermatology*.

This book covers all the focused and yet important topics on skin and hormones by experts of Indian dermatologists and physicians. It includes the main topic of interest, which is polycystic ovarian disease, out of which is a very important clinical topic—*polycystic ovarian disease* (PCOD), with many controversial investigations and lines of management. Through this book, doctors can learn to approach such complicated cases of PCOD.

Chapters also provide information about other common yet less discussed hormonal issues such as diabetes, thyroid disease, obesity affecting skin, and what signs and symptoms should be looked for in such patients for early diagnosis and treatment. Hence, this book offers assistance to dermatologists, consulting physicians, postgraduates, and interns in the holistic understanding and practical management of common as well as other miscellaneous issues like diet and hormones and urticaria and hormones.

This would add value to all the chapters, which are easy to understand with simple language, clinical pictures, and graphs.

Gurugram, India — Naresh Trehan

Preface

Hormonal diseases are known to affect Skin Health. This book covers all the focused and yet important topics on skin and hormones by experts of Indian dermatologists and physicians. It majorly covers various important aspects of most common hormonal disease—Polycystic Ovarian Disease (PCOD), i.e. its pathogenesis, investigations, and individual clinical features with their line of management.

Chapters also provide information about other common yet less discussed hormonal issues such as diabetes, thyroid disease, obesity affecting skin, and what signs and symptoms should be looked for in such patients for early diagnosis and treatment.

Hence, this book offers assistance to dermatologists, consulting physicians, postgraduates, and interns in the holistic understanding and practical management of common as well as other miscellaneous issues like diet and hormones and urticaria and hormones.

Gurgaon, India — Ramanjit Singh
Gurgaon, Haryana, India — Nidhi Sharma

Contents

Chapter 1
Overview of Endocrinology

Sunil Mishra and Gazal Bakshi

The endocrine and integumentary systems interact with each other through various mechanisms. Dysregulation of endocrine hormones often results in clinically significant dermatologic manifestation. These cutaneous lesions can serve as markers of endocrine disease or vice versa. The dermatologic manifestations can be specific to the underlying endocrinological disorder and can help in the early diagnosis and treatment. Whenever possible, it is crucial to identify the underlying endocrine disorder to provide corrective treatment for skin symptoms rather than providing just the symptomatic treatment [1].

1.1 Disorder of the Hypothalamic-Pituitary Axis

1.1.1 Acromegaly

Acromegaly is a chronic disorder caused by growth hormone hypersecretion. GH circulates and stimulates the production of IGF-1 which in large part mediates the somatic and metabolic effects of GH. Excessive secretion of growth hormone leads to increased production of IGF-1, leading to a multisystem disease characterized by somatic overgrowth, multiple comorbidities, premature mortality, and physical disfigurement [2].

S. Mishra (✉) · G. Bakshi
Division of Endocrinology and Diabetes, Medanta, The Medicity, Gurugram, Gurugram, Haryana, India

R. Singh, N. Sharma (eds.), *A Guide to Hormonal Dermatology*,
https://doi.org/10.1007/978-981-99-7715-4_1

1.1.1.1 Dermatologic Manifestations

1. Facial features

   Coarsening of the chin, nose, and supraorbital ridges as well as prognathism, macroglossia, macrocheilia, and gingival hyperplasia manifest due to facial thickening and edema. These patients have a typical melancholic expression because of pronounced nasolabial groove, increased size, redness, and wrinkling of the forehead. The increase in dermal collagen and consequent buckling and coarse furrowing of skin on the scalp causes cutis verticis gyrata [3].
2. Hand and feet:

   There is a disproportionate enlargement of fingertips, leading to a drumstick-like appearance of fingers and toes.
3. Other features:

   These patients may develop acanthosis nigricans. Increased production by sebaceous and sweat glands manifests as oily skin and hyperhidrosis, respectively. Involvement of the hair and nails can result in hypertrichosis and platonychia respectively [4].

1.1.2 Hypopituitarism

It is characterized by a relative or absolute deficiency of one or more pituitary hormones like ACTH, Prolactin, luteinizing hormone, Follicle stimulating hormone, Thyroid stimulating hormone, Growth hormone and Antidiuretic hormone (Table 1.1).

Table 1.1 Systemic and dermatologic manifestations of hypopituitarism [5]

Hormone	Major clinical manifestations of deficiency	Major dermatologic manifestations of deficiency
ACTH	Fatigue, anorexia, nausea, hypotension, hypoglycemia, hypothermia	Skin hypopigmentation, decreased skin turgor, dry skin, auricular calcification
TSH	Fatigue, constipation, weight gain, cold intolerance, dry, rough, and scaly skin GH impaired quality of life; altered musculoskeletal composition, impaired cardiac function, increased cardiovascular risk	Dry, rough and scaly skin
GH	Impaired quality of life; altered musculoskeletal composition; impaired cardiac function; increased cardiovascular risk	Thin and dry skin; fat deposition in chest and abdomen
FSH/LH	Amenorrhea; decreased libido; impotence; infertility	In men—decreased facial folds, fine wrinkling around eyes and mouth, absent facial and body hair, smooth scrotum; in women—dry, atrophic, and pruritic skin; wrinkling as above

1.2 Thyroid Related Disorders

1.2.1 Hyperthyroidism

It is most commonly seen in Graves' disease and other causes including thyroiditis, toxic multinodular goiter, toxic adenoma, and exogenous thyroid hormone use. Graves' disease is an autoimmune thyroid disorder due to autoantibodies to the thyrotropin receptors.

The cutaneous manifestations seen among patients with Graves' disease are due to excess thyroid hormone and certain extrathyroidal manifestations occur due to the effect of thyroid stimulating immunoglobulins on thyrotropin receptors found in the skin and connective tissue [1].

1.2.1.1 Dermatological Manifestations

1. Thyroid dermopathy

   It presents as pretibial myxedema resulting in flesh-coloured or yellowish-brown, raised skin lesions overlying a non-pitting thickening and induration at sites like the anterior tibia followed by the dorsum of the feet and the toes and areas subjected to repeated trauma, surgical scars, and burns. It can occur in 4% of individuals. In advanced stages, these lesions may become hyperkeratotic, nodular or fungating [6].

   Excess hormone leads to the overstimulation of adrenergic receptors and causes increased body temperature and hyperhidrosis and manifests as soft, warm, and moist skin. Hyperhidrosis can be observed in palms and soles [6]. The epidermis is found to be thin but not atrophic as in Cushing syndrome.
2. Hairs

   Scalp hair often has a downy texture. Diffuse scalp hair thinning can be noted, although the degree of hair loss has no correlation with disease severity.
3. Nails

   Onycholysis, that is loosening of the nails from the nail bed, can be seen. Plummer's nail with upturned nail plate due to the pink coloured proximal portion and white opaque coloured distal portion of nail plate. It is most likely to be first seen on the fourth fingernail [6].

   Approximately 0.1–1% present with a rare manifestation of Graves' disease, thyroid acropachy. It is characterized by the triad of digital clubbing, acral swelling, and diaphyseal proliferation of the periosteum in acral and distal long bones. It is more common in adults, and only rarely reported in pediatric patients [7].

   Less common cutaneous manifestations of hyperthyroidism include generalized pruritus, eczematous dermatitis, chronic urticaria and dermographism.

1.2.2 Hypothyroidism

The most common aetiology for the development of hypothyroidism is Hashimoto's thyroiditis or chronic lymphocytic thyroiditis. Other causes of hypothyroidism are iodine deficiency iatrogenic following 131I treatment, post thyroidectomy, or due to various drugs like lithium, bexarotene, or interferon.

1.2.2.1 Dermatological Manifestations

1. Skin

   Over 80% of individuals with primary hypothyroidism often have cold, mottled, dry skin. The epidermis is thin, rough, and hyperkeratotic giving a scaly appearance [8].

   Patients with secondary hypothyroidism often demonstrate a fine wrinkling of the skin that imparts a parchment-like quality.

   Carotenemia due to reduced hepatic conversion of beta carotene to vitamin A, can deposit in the stratum corneum and manifest as a yellowing of the skin. It commonly affects the palms, soles, and nasolabial folds. The absence of scleral involvement can differentiate it from jaundice.

   In severe cases of hypothyroidism, the accumulation of mucopolysaccharides can cause myxedema. The hands, face, pretibial, and periorbital areas are most commonly affected resulting in a non-pitting oedema with the broadening of the nose, thickening of the lips, and macroglossia. As there is decreased sympathetic stimulation the outer third of the eyebrow can be lost and ptosis can occur. Facial expressions may be blunted and can make it difficult to interpret emotions [9].
2. Hairs

   Hairs are usually rough and brittle due to reduced sebum secretion. Around 50% of patients with hypothyroidism may have diffuse or partial alopecia, often including genital and beard hair. On the other way round, hypertrichosis of the back and shoulders in children can be a sign of hypothyroidism.
3. Nails

   They can be brittle and striated.

   Other autoimmune conditions can also be associated like dermatitis herpetiformis, alopecia areata, vitiligo, and autoimmune urticaria.

1.3 Disorders of the Adrenal Gland

1.3.1 Cushing Syndrome

It is caused by hypercortisolemia and occurs due to pituitary (Cushing's disease) or ectopic hypersecretion of adrenocorticotropic hormone (ACTH), adrenal overproduction of cortisol, or iatrogenic administration of glucocorticoids. Due to excessive amounts of glucocorticoids, there can be decreased proliferation of keratinocytes and dermal fibroblasts. These changes decrease the formation of collagen and other components of the extracellular matrix and contribute to skin atrophy and fragility [9].

1.3.1.1 Dermatologic Manifestations

Deposition of adipose tissue in characteristic locations contributes to the Cushingoid appearance causing moon facies, dorsocervical fat pad appearing as a buffalo hump, supraclavicular fat pad, and behind the orbit. The subcutaneous tissue loss causes easy bruisability and delayed wound healing. The epidermal and dermal loss of tissue on the elbows and dorsum of the hands results in 'Cigarette paper' skin.

Due to redistribution and enlargement of body mass, the fragile skin further stretches and subcutaneous blood vessels become easily visible, appearing as purple striae. The violaceous, thick (>1 cm in diameter) dehiscent striae of Cushing syndrome can be distinguished from the pink silver, thin striae observed in puberty, obesity, and pregnancy.

Other changes can manifest as acanthosis nigricans due to metabolic changes or hyperpigmentation in ACTH dependent forms.

1.3.2 Primary Adrenal Insufficiency

It is a condition characterized by the failure of the adrenal glands to produce cortisol. The common etiologies are Addison's disease, autoimmune adrenalitis; infections like tuberculosis, histoplasmosis etc.; storage disorders like sarcoidosis etc.

The loss of negative feedback on the hypothalamic-pituitary axis occurs due to decreased cortisol production. This increases the production of corticotropin releasing hormone and thereby, proopiomelanocortin, a precursor of ACTH, melanocyte-stimulating hormone (MSH), and others. Elevated levels of MSH consequently trigger melanin synthesis by epidermal melanocytes via melanocortin type 1 receptor [10].

1.3.2.1 Dermatologic Manifestations

Hyperpigmentation

It is observed in almost all adult patients and 67% of pediatric patients. It is most prominent in sun-exposed areas as well as areas of trauma, pressure and recent scars. Other frequently affected body parts include the axilla, areolas, perineum, and palmar creases and mucosal surfaces involving the tongue, inner surface of the lip, as well as buccal and gingival mucosa. In addition, patients may notice darkening of existing nevi [1].

Vitiligo, caused by the autoimmune destruction of dermal melanocytes, occurs in 10–20% of individuals with autoimmune adrenalitis [7].

Women with Addison's disease may experience a loss of axillary and pubic hair due to affected adrenal androgen production.

1.3.3 Other Causes of Adrenal Insufficiency and Associated Skin Manifestations

Waterhouse-Friderichsen syndrome is adrenal hemorrhage (usually bilateral) caused by severe bacterial infection associated most commonly with meningococcemia. The primary dermatologic finding is the presence of petechial eruptions on the trunk progressing to purpuric rash [7].

Polyglandular autoimmune syndrome type 1 is a rare immunodeficiency syndrome due to mutation of the autoimmune regulator gene. It is characterized by chronic mucocutaneous candidiasis, hypoparathyroidism, adrenal insufficiency, and primary hypogonadism [7].

1.3.3.1 Skin Manifestations

A characteristic feature of APECED is chronic mucocutaneous candidiasis. Affecting all patients by the age of 40 and can be oral, gastrointestinal, or genitourinary. APECED is often accompanied by autoimmune disorders like dental enamel hypoplasia, keratoconjunctivitis, alopecia, or vitiligo.

1.3.4 Pseudohypoaldosteronism

It is a syndrome characterized by resistance to the action of aldosterone. Pseudohypoaldosteronism type I has two forms. The autosomal dominant form is caused by a mutation in the NR3C2 gene encoding mineralocorticoid receptors specific to the kidney. The autosomal recessive form results from loss of activity in the epithelial sodium channel affecting all aldosterone targets, including the distal nephron.

1.3.4.1 Dermatological Manifestations

Miliaria rubra, a pustular, erythematous skin lesion, has been described in infants with pseudohypoaldosteronism type I. The mechanism of occurrence of these lesions is proposed to be due to the obstruction of eccrine sweat glands caused by excess excretion of sodium that tends to occur during hyponatremic crises. The lesions improve with the correction of electrolyte abnormalities [11].

1.4 Disorder of Parathyroid Hormone

Primary hyperparathyroidism leads to hypercalcemia via the overproduction of parathyroid hormone.

1.4.1 Dermatological Manifestations

Rarely, Benign nodular calcification is a form of calcinosis cutis that may occur due to metastatic calcification characterized by indurated white papules or plaques located in the subcutaneous tissue. These tend to be located near the joints.

The most severe skin manifestation of hyperparathyroidism is calciphylaxis, or calcification of blood vessels supplying cutaneous tissue. It presents as mottled skin lesions resembling livedo reticularis which later becomes painful and undergoes necrosis followed by the development of an overlying eschar. Sepsis may occur due to bacterial superinfection of these lesions [12].

1.5 Disorder of the Endocrine Pancreas

1.5.1 Diabetes Mellitus

Different specific and nonspecific (related to metabolic changes) cutaneous manifestations are observed. These include recurrent cutaneous fungal or bacterial infections, necrobiosis lipoidica diabeticorum (0.3–1.6%), diabetic bullae (0.5%), and autoimmune-related cutaneous disorders such as vitiligo. Diabetic dermopathy is the most common dermatological finding, in up to 70% of adult patients with diabetes [13].

1.5.1.1 Dermatologic Manifestations

1. Acanthosis nigricans:

   Acanthosis nigricans is a diffuse, velvety thickening and hyperpigmentation of the skin associated with T2DM. It usually involves axillae, neck, inframammary folds, inguinal folds, and perineum. Along with acanthosis nigricans, it is common to see skin tags or acrochordons [14].

   Hyperinsulinemia in type 2 diabetes mellitus cause increased signaling via IGF-1 receptors, present in cultured fibroblasts and keratinocytes. The affinity of these receptors to bind IGF-1 is 100–1000 times greater than insulin. Thus, the insulin-dependent increase in IGF-1 and activation of signaling pathway promotes cellular growth and differentiation causing acanthosis [15].

2. Cutaneous infections:

   There is an increased predisposition to infections like staphylococcal pyodermas, candidiasis, erythrasma, and dermatophyte infections [16].
3. Necrobiosis lipoidica diabeticorum (NLD)

   It has a predisposition for women and patients who are insulin-dependent. Around 75% of necrobiosis lipoidica diabeticorum cases occur in patients with or who may develop diabetes mellitus with predilection towards anterior or lateral lower leg. The lesions are varied from well demarcated oval to irregularly shaped. They have indurated plaques with yellow pigmentation at the centre and red-brown or violaceous pigmentation at the periphery. Later, the centre may become atrophic with superficial telangiectasias or can ulcerate in up to 33% of patients [16].
4. Diabetic dermopathy

   It is the most common skin manifestation of diabetes and affects up to 70% of adult diabetic patients. The common involved site is the anterior shin where it manifests as irregularly shaped, light brown macules and patches. Upon resolution, patients may develop areas of atrophy or scarring.
5. Scleredema adultorum

   It is more common in adult patients and rarely reported in children just like dermopathy. It presents as painless, non-pitting swelling starting from the lateral and posterior neck and can later spread to the anterior neck, shoulders, face, and upper torso. Patients with T1DM are at slightly higher risk.

   Other cutaneous manifestations in patients with DM include carotenemia, lipodystrophy, hemochromatosis, and xanthomatosis secondary to hyperlipidemia.

1.5.2 Glucagonoma

It is a malignant tumour of the alpha cell of the pancreas which secretes the hormone glucagon. The glucagonoma syndrome is characterized by the triad of glucagonoma, diabetes mellitus, and a skin lesion known as necrolytic migratory erythema [17].

1.5.2.1 Dermatological Manifestations

Necrolytic migratory erythema is the major dermatologic manifestation of glucagonoma, occurring in almost all patients during the course of the disease. The initial dermatologic eruption is characterized by erythema that progresses to form painful, pruritic bullae or vesicular lesions over the course of 7–14 days. These can later burst and spread outwards causing hyperpigmentation and crusting of the affected areas. The commonly involved sites are in the groin and then spread to the extremities, thighs, buttocks, and perineum. The perioral area may also be affected. Superinfection, either bacterial or fungal, is common. In areas exposed to constant friction, they become lichenified or may resemble psoriasis. These lesions may also occur in areas exposed to trauma, a phenomenon known as koebnerization. A biopsy of the lesion is needed to confirm the diagnosis of NME [17].

1.6 Disorder of Androgen Excess

1.6.1 Polycystic Ovarian Syndrome

PCOS is one of the most common disorders associated with androgen excess. Various others are congenital adrenal hyperplasia as well as an ovarian or adrenal tumour. PCOS is characterized by evidence of hyperandrogenism and chronic anovulation in the absence of any pituitary or adrenal pathology.

1.6.1.1 Dermatologic Manifestations

1. Hirsutism

   It is defined as excess terminal hair growth in a male-pattern distribution including the beard area (face and neck), back, chest and lower abdomen [7]. Hyperandrogenism can cause an increase in the hair fibres circumference and prolongs the anagen phase of hair growth in the beard, axillary, and pubic regions whereas androgen levels do not correlate with the quantity of hair growth [18].
2. Acne vulgaris

   Androgen excess is considered in patients with moderate to severe nodulocystic acne which are resistant to conventional therapies or may recur after treatment.
3. Virilization

   It is characterized by a deepening of the voice, muscle hypertrophy, reduction in breast size, clitoromegaly, and androgenetic alopecia. Individuals with hair loss have a gradual thinning of the hair mostly affecting the vertex and upper biparietal region of the scalp with preservation of the anterior hairline [18].
4. Acanthosis nigricans

1.7 Hereditary Endocrine Syndromes

1.7.1 Multiple Endocrine Neoplasia (MEN) Syndromes

1.7.1.1 MEN1

It is an autosomal dominant disease that results from the inactivation of the menin tumour suppressor gene. It is characterized by parathyroid adenomas, pancreatic islet tumours, and tumours of the anterior pituitary gland.

Angiofibromas, appearing as flesh colored, pink, or red papules with smooth and shiny surfaces, are the most common cutaneous manifestation of MEN1. Other common dermatologic findings include lipomas, café-au-lait spots, and collagenomas. Collagenomas are described as "skin-colored to slightly hypopigmented, dome-shaped, well-circumscribed, firm, round to oval papules" and tend to occur on the upper portion of the torso, neck, and shoulders. Glucagonoma occur in only 3% patients with MEN 1 but is typically associated with necrolytic migratory erythema [19].

1.7.1.2 MEN 2

It occurs due to activating mutations in the RET protooncogene.

MEN 2A: The most significant dermatologic manifestation is lichen amyloidosis occurring usually on extensor surfaces of the upper back and extremities. Lesions are gray brown, intensely pruritic, hyperkeratotic papules [1].

MEN2B: Mucosal neuromas commonly occur on the lips, tongue, eyelids, and conjunctiva in the fifth decade involving the anterior one-third of the tongue commonly. Ganglioneuromas can cause a diffuse, fleshy projection of lips. These patients have increased incidence of café-au-lait macules.

1.8 Neurofibromatosis 1

It is an autosomal-dominant caused by a mutation in the neurofibromin gene. Mosaicism occurring due to postzygotic somatic mutation causes unilateral cutaneous findings. Endocrine implications of NF1 can include growth hormone deficiency, growth hormone excess, precocious puberty, gynecomastia, and/or pheochromocytoma.

1.8.1 Skin Manifestations

1. Neurofibromas are the key dermatologic manifestation of NF1 and are present in >99% of patients. Schwann cells with a mutation in NF-1 gene, secrete stem cell factors that drive mast cells into the lesion, which further express TGFβ leading to the proliferation of collagen and cellular growth and tumour formation. They can be subcategorized into cutaneous (focal or diffuse), subcutaneous, plexiform (nodular or diffuse), and spinal. The invagination on pressing the lesion called the "Buttonhole" sign is pathognomonic.
2. Plexiform neurofibromas are specifically found among NF1 (30–50%) patients in the adolescent age group. They follow a nerve fascicle, where the overlying skin can become rough and hyperpigmented and their number may increase with age and pregnancy.

3. Café-au-lait macules are hyperpigmented, well-demarcated, round macules present in >99% of patients; these may manifest at birth and their number stabilizes with age such that more than 6 café-au-lait macules are highly suggestive of NF1.
4. Freckling is pathognomonic. It presents in 3–4 years of life as the small (1–4 mm), clustered pigmentary macules of the axillary region and groin or areas with minimal to no sun exposure. They are present in >85% of patients and can be increased by friction, temperature or moisture.

1.9 Von Hippel Lindau

It is an autosomal-dominant disease associated with the mutation of the VHL tumour suppressor gene. Hemangioblastomas, renal cell carcinoma, Pancreatic neuroendocrine tumours, Pheochromocytoma can be associated.

1.9.1 Skin Manifestations

These are relatively uncommon and include nonspecific cutaneous hemangiomas and café-au-lait spots.

1.10 Conclusion

Skin is the mirror of various conditions defining the health of a patient. While few dermatological manifestations can be pathognomonic of the underlying endocrine disorders (e.g., NME in patients with glucagonoma), some are part of the diagnostic criteria (e.g., MEN1) and rest can be nonspecific and may require a more careful evaluation. Hence, skin can be considered to be a screen displaying underlying endocrine disorders. Healthcare providers should be able to recognize these disorders, associate them with the underlying endocrine problem, and perform further workup to make a final diagnosis.

References

1. Lause M, Kamboj A, Faith EF. Dermatologic manifestations of endocrine disorders. Transl Pediatr. 2017;6(4):300–12.
2. Katznelson L, Laws ER Jr, Melmed S, Molitch ME, Murad MH, Utz A, Wass JA. Acromegaly: an endocrine society clinical practice guideline. J Clin Endocrinol Metabol. 2014;99(11):3933–51.
3. Shareef S, Horowitz D, Kaliyadan F. Cutis Verticis Gyrata. In: StatPearls [Internet]. Treasure Island: StatPearls Publishing; 2022.

4. Ben-Shlomo A, Melmed S. Skin manifestations in acromegaly. Clin Dermatol. 2006;24(4):256–9.
5. Geller JL, Braunstein GD. Dermatologic manifestations of hypopituitarism. Clin Dermatol. 2006;24(4):266–75.
6. Raj R, Elshimy G, Mishra R, Jha N, Joseph V, Bratman R, Tella SH, Correa R. Dermatologic manifestations of endocrine disorders. Cureus. 2021;13(9):e18327.
7. Melmed S, Koenig R, Rosen C, Auchus R, Goldfine A. Williams textbook of endocrinology. 14th ed. New Delhi: Elsevier; 2020.
8. Alcázar Lázaro V, Aguilar MA. Alteraciones dermatológicas asociadasa hipotiroidismo. Endocrinol Nutr. 2013;60(6):345–7.
9. Stratakis CA. Skin manifestations of Cushing's syndrome. Rev Endocr Metab Disorders. 2016;17:283–6.
10. Thody AJ. α-MSH and the regulation of melanocyte function. Ann N Y Acad Sci. 1999;885(1):217–29.
11. Urbatsch A, Paller AS. Pustular miliaria rubra: a specific cutaneous finding of type I pseudohypoaldosteronism. Pediatr Dermatol. 2002;19(4):317–9.
12. Fuleihan GE, Rubeiz N. Dermatologic manifestations of parathyroid-related disorders. Clin Dermatol. 2006;24(4):281–8.
13. Rongioletti F. Pancreas disease and diabetes mellitus. In: Clinical and pathological aspects of skin diseases in endocrine, metabolic, nutritional and deposition disease. New York: Springer; 2010. p. 11–25.
14. Brady MF, Rawla P. Acanthosis nigricans. In: StatPearls [Internet]. Treasure Island: StatPearls Publishing; 2024.
15. Kapoor S. Diagnosis and treatment of acanthosis nigricans. Skinmed. 2010;8(3):161–4.
16. Labib A, Rosen J, Yosipovitch G. Skin manifestations of diabetes mellitus. In: Feingold KR, Anawalt B, Boyce A, editors. Endotext [Internet]. South Dartmouth: MDText.com, Inc.; 2022.
17. Foss MG, Ferrer-Bruker SJ. Necrolytic migratory erythema. In: StatPearls [Internet]. Treasure Island: StatPearls Publishing; 2021.
18. Abusailik MA, Muhanna AM, Almuhisen AA, Alhasanat AM, Alshamaseen AM, Mustafa SM, Nawaiseh MB. Cutaneous manifestation of polycystic ovary syndrome. Dermatol Rep. 2021;13(2):8799.
19. Vidal A, Iglesias MJ, Fernández B, Fonseca E, Cordido F. Cutaneous lesions associated to multiple endocrine neoplasia syndrome type 1. J Eur Acad Dermatol Venereol. 2008;22(7):835–8.

Chapter 2
Obesity and Skin

Nidhi Sharma, Priyadarshini Sahu, and Amalia Tsiatoura

2.1 Introduction

Obesity is one of the major public health problems worldwide, which has been increasing with a rapid rate in past two decades. Objective way to define obesity is BMI (body mass index). ≥ 30 kg/m^2 BMI is considered as obesity [1].

2.2 Effect of Obesity on Skin Pathophysiology

Obesity is a complex condition that affects every part of the human body, including the skin. It's important to note that 60–70% of obese people have various skin changes [2]. It alters skin physiology, collagen structure, and wound healing due to an elevated body mass index. It also affects sebaceous and sweat glands, circulation, and lymphatic systems. Common skin issues associated with obesity include acanthosis nigricans, acrochordons, keratosis pilaris, striae distensae, cellulite, and plantar hyperkeratosis. Obesity can lead to metabolic effects like hyperandrogenism and gout, which affect the skin. Moreover, it increases the risk of skin infections, inflammatory conditions, and chronic dermatoses like psoriasis and rosacea. Understanding these skin changes is vital for early diagnosis and appropriate treatment [3].

N. Sharma
Skin Health clinic, Gurugram, Haryana, India

P. Sahu (✉)
Consultant Dermatologist, Department of Telemedicine, PGIMER, Chandigarh, India

A. Tsiatoura
Cosmetic Derma Medicine Center, Athens, Greece
e-mail: amalia.tsiatoura@cosmeticdermamedicine.gr

R. Singh, N. Sharma (eds.), *A Guide to Hormonal Dermatology*,
https://doi.org/10.1007/978-981-99-7715-4_2

1. **Skin barrier**:

   Obesity affects the barrier integrity and leads to altered trans-epidermal water loss (TEWL) and xerosis. In morbidly obese patients, hydration of stratum corneum changes, resulting in higher TEWL secondary to profuse sweating. Increased TEWL leads to xerosis [4].
2. **Collagen structure and wound healing**:

   Obesity is associated with impaired wound healing due to altered collagen structure. In obese patients, increase in skin surface area is more as compared to collagen deposition, resulting in decrease in mechanical strength of skin. Further obesity is accompanied with leptin resistance and leptin helps in wound healing, which further results in impaired wound healing [5]. Thus, obesity contributes to the pathological cycle of impaired wound healing.
3. **Sweat glands**:

   Obese patients have thick layers of subcutaneous fat and large skin folds, that leads to profuse sweating. Increased subcutaneous fat augments moisture and frictional component of skin. This produces humid environment, which exacerbates local inflammation, predisposing to dermatoses such as candida species, dermatophytosis, intertrigo and further leads to secondary bacterial infection. Obesity leads to intertrigo and diabetes, which promote bacterial growth and further bromhidrosis [6].
4. **Sebaceous glands and sebum production**:

   In obese patients' sebum production is increased due to elevated levels of androgens, growth hormones, insulin and insulin like growth factor. All these factors, play a pivotal role in development of acne.
5. **Lymphatic and Circulatory changes**:

   The primary cause of microvascular dysfunction is obesity, that results in microangiopathy and hypertension. This leads to chronic venous diseases like varicose veins and ulceration. Venous insufficiency can be associated with Lipodermatosclerosis; a chronic form of panniculitis [7]. In addition, obesity can affect lymphatic flow, which results in lymphedema, resulting in increased risk of infection.

2.3 Common Skin Changes Associated with Obesity

2.3.1 Acanthosis Nigricans (AN)

Clinical presentation—It is characterised by symmetrical pigmentation with coarse thickened skin covered by small papillomatous elevations, giving it a velvety texture. As there is increase in thickness, skin lines get further accentuated and surface becomes rugose and mamillated. It is usually asymptomatic in nature and sometimes it may be pruritic. It usually affects back, sides of neck, groin, axillae, popliteal and ante-cubital area.

Pathogenesis—It is primarily associated with obesity and type 2 diabetes mellitus. Both these condition leads to hyperinsulinemia. Hyperinsulinemia can increase blood levels of insulin like growth factor 1 (IGF-1) and directly activate IGF-1 receptors on skin cells. Binding of IGFRs stimulates proliferation of keratinocytes and fibroblast leading to AN. Other contributing factors include Tyrosine kinase receptors like epidermal growth factor receptors and Fibroblast growth factor receptors [8].

Diagnosis is usually clinical and histopathology is needed only in case of doubt.

Treatment—In case of obesity related AN, weight loss must be the first line of therapy. Exercise, diet and behavioural modification is the mainstay of weight reduction. Further topical treatment includes topical retinoids, keratolytics, calcipotriol, chemical peeling with trichloroacetic acid, and LASERs. Systemic treatment includes retinoids like isotretinoin and insulin sensitizers like metformin [9].

2.3.2 Keratosis Pilaris

Clinical features—It is characterized by spiny keratotic papules with surrounding erythema. It usually affects the extensor surface of proximal extremities i.e., extensor surface of proximal arm, thigh and checks. It is usually associated with many conditions such as obesity, diabetes mellitus, malnutrition, atopic dermatitis and ichthyosis vulgaris.

Pathogenesis—The pathophysiology still remains an enigma. The most accepted theory suggest that it is a disorder of follicular epithelial keratinization triggering an infundibular plug formation. This keratotic plug results in erythema and scaling around the follicular opening along with coiled hairs within the lesion [10]. Diagnosis is mainly based on history and clinical examination and biopsy is not required in most of the cases.

Treatment—The condition usually improves with time but several treatment options are available. General measures include maintaining adequate hygiene, using hypoallergic soap and refraining from manipulating the papules. Topical treatment includes emollients and topical keratolytic agents. Topical keratolytic includes topical retinoids, 6% salicylic acid lotion, 20% urea cream and vitamin D3 derivatives i.e., 0.01% tazarotene. When applied at night time, lesions fade within 2 weeks and after 4–8 weeks KP gets resolved. Chemical peeling i.e., 70% glycolic peel has also been used to improve the appearance. Some dermatologists have also used LASERs especially pulse dye laser, Nd-YAG laser, alexandrite laser and fractional CO_2 laser and found it be quite successful [11].

2.3.3 Achrocordons

Clinical features—It is also known as Skin tag. It is usually benign in nature and characterized by cutaneous growth seen as skin coloured or brown coloured growth that are often pedunculated and attached to a fleshy stalk. It is seen more commonly in individuals suffering from diabetes, obesity, metabolic syndrome and patients having family history of skin tags. Generally, it is asymptomatic but sometimes it can result in bleeding or itching if caught in clothing or jewellery. Acrochordons when seen in large number it forms a necklace like configuration around the neck and known as "molluscum pendulum necklace sign". It has a reported incidence of 50–60% in general population [12].

Pathogenesis—In obese patients, frequent irritation of skin is the prime cause. Some clinicians also believe that it is due to normal aging process of skin that results in loss of elasticity. Elevated levels of progesterone, estrogen, other female sex hormones and elevated levels of human growth hormone can also potentiate skin tag development. Both Epidermal growth factor (EGF) and alpha tissue growth factor can also be risk factors for acrochordon [13].

Treatment—It can be easily diagnosed by clinical examination. Removal of skin tag is the mainstay of treatment. It can be removed with radio-cautery, snip excision and cryotherapy. Small skin tags can be removed with lasers especially nanosecond Q-switched Nd:YAG or CO_2 laser.

2.3.4 Striae Distensae (SD)

Clinical features—It is also known as Stretch mark. It is characterised by linear scar which develop as a result of excessive stretching of skin. Initial lesions of SD are smooth, raised, irritable and erythematous to bluish in colour. It is also known as Striae rubra. As the lesion progress, it flattens and becomes pale and irregular with finely wrinkled surface. These flatten pale linear scar is known as striae alba. Thigh, buttocks and breast in girls and lumbosacral region and outer aspects of thigh in boys are most commonly affected site [14].

The diagnosis is usually start-forward without any specific investigation.

Pathogenesis—Exact etiopathogenesis is still not clear. The primary pathology is the altered dermal connective tissue framework involving components of extra-cellular matrix (ECM) especially elastin, fibronectin, fibrillin and collagen. Initially, elastic fibres undergo elastolysis and degranulation of mast cells. Low expression of fibronectin and collagen genes in the affected tissue or high amount of rigid cross-linked collagen, makes the connective tissue more prone to stress rupture.

Treatment—General measures include prevention of development of stretch marks by avoidance of brisk weight gain or loss; particularly in high-risk group i.e., adolescents, athletes and pregnant women. Exercise and diet modification plays a prime role in reduction SD in early days. Various topical agents such as tretinoin, hyaluronic acid, trofolastin, silicone, pirfenidone, ascorbic acid, glycolic acid, olive oil, almond oil, coconut oil and bio-oil. Various procedures include lasers (i.e., fractional CO_2, Er:YAG, and Nd:YAG laser), Microneedling radiofrequency, microdermabrasion, platelet rich plasma (PRP), and chemical peeling.

2.3.5 *Cellulite*

Clinical features—Cellulite is a painless skin condition presented with dimpling and denting of the skin surface, giving it an orange peel appearance. It is a common condition occurring in about 80–90% of post-pubertal women of all races. Mostly it occurs in areas with greater fat storage like buttocks, abdomen and thighs [15].

Pathogenesis—The etiopathogenesis is not well-established. Environmental, hormonal and genetic plays an important role in development of cellulite. Environmental factors include improper lifestyle and consumption of alcohol. Hormonal factors such as increase oestrogen levels may contribute to formation of cellulite. Men are affected rarely, due to low androgen levels. Condition causing low androgens levels such as Klinefelter's syndrome, hypogonadism, anti-androgen therapy for prostate and after castration may also lead to its formation. It may be associated with obesity, insulin resistance and increase cardiovascular risk.

Treatment—Lifestyle modification is the important step in genetically predisposed individual and prevention of cellulite worsening. Proper diet with low sodium and fat content, exercise and restricting alcohol and smoking are recommended for patients with cellulite. Topical preparations containing caffeine, methylxanthines, retinol, alpha bisabolol, carica papaya extract, other plant extracts, vegetable oils, ascorbic acid, squalene and urea. These cocktail preparation works on decreasing lipogenesis, improvement in microcirculation, increase lipolysis, increase in extracellular matrix synthesis and integrity, and decrease oxidation and inflammation. Other treatment modalities include subcision, oral collagen peptide massage, extracorporeal shock wave therapy, radiofrequency, dermal fillers, collagenase clostridium histolyticum, carboxytherapy, ultrasound, laser and light devices can also be used. Thus, combination of treatment is more beneficial as compared to a single modality of treatment.

2.3.6 *Plantar Hyperkeratosis*

Clinical features—It presents as thickened skin over heel, foot arch and great toe giving an appearance of horseshoe. So, it is known as horseshoe-like hyperkeratosis. This may be due decrease in plantar arch, and increased gravity load of heels due to obesity [16].

Pathogenesis—This may be due to high pressure over the bony prominence of soles and weight bearing areas especially heals and plantar arch, leading to decrease in plantar arch and its hyperkeratosis.

Treatment—Topical keratolytic agents i.e., urea and salicylic based creams can be used to reduce the thickening. Additionally, treatment options for plantar hyperkeratosis may encompass physical therapy, exercises to enhance foot function, alleviate pressure, and, in severe cases, surgical procedures. If not addressed, this condition can lead to complications such as ulcers and infections, which are especially problematic for people with obesity because their skin's integrity is compromised.

2.3.7 Skin Infections

Clinical features—Obesity increases risk of skin infections and also negatively affect its outcome. Incidence of various bacterial and fungal infection increases. Bacterial infection includes furunculosis, erysipelas, cellulitis, erythrasma, folliculitis, necrotizing fasciitis and gas gangrene increased in obese patients. Fungal infections such as candidiasis, candida folliculitis, intertrigo, hand and feet paronychia, onychomycosis and tinea cruris are more prevalent. Further due to recurrent bacterial infections secondary to impaired lymphatics results in elephantiasis nostras verrucosa [2].

Pathogenesis—Decreased cell-mediated immune response, proinflammatory state in obese patient, and inability to maintain adequate levels of hygiene might exacerbate this problem.

Treatment—Management can be done according to the etiology.

2.4 Rare Skin Conditions Associated with Obesity

2.4.1 Keratosis Follicularis Squamosa (Dohi; KFS)

Clinical features—KFS is a keratinizing disorder, clinically characterized by 3–10 mm diameter scaly patches with brownish colour follicular plugs in the centre and slightly raised margin as compared to the underlying epidermis. It is scattered on the trunk, thigh and buttock. It is well-recognised entity in Japan and rarely reported in other countries. It was originally described as 'lotus leave on water' [17].

Pathogenesis—The exact pathogenesis is yet to be fully elucidated. Bacterial infection, genetics, irritation by clothes and hormonal imbalance have been proposed as the pathogenic factors. The novel locus for KPS on chromosome is 7p14.3-7p12.1. Some cases have also shown Gram positive cocci in the dilated follicles and coagulase negative staphylococcus in the biopsied specimen. Histopathology shows dilated hair follicle with follicular plug surrounded by lamellar orthohyperkeratosis.

Treatment—In most of cases, it is treated with minocycline. One case has shown efficacy with roxithromycin. Topical urea, vitamin D ointment and salicylic acid has been tried as treatment without long lasting effect. Long term follow-up of the disease is poor.

2.4.2 Adiposis Dolorosa/Dercum Disease (DD)

Clinical features—It is a rare disease that typically presents as multiple, painful subcutaneous adipose tissue deposits of variable size and location. The pain is burning and searing. Pain can be severe, chronic (>3 months) and is disabling. The skin over the affected area is unchanged. It predominantly affects post-menopausal women. The painful deposits of dercum disease are small and quite difficult to palpate in comparison to nodule of lipoma, that can achieve large size and mass [18].

Pathogenesis—autosomal dominant inheritance with incomplete penetrance has been suggested for the disease. It may be associated with overweight and obesity, weakness or fatigue and a number of psychiatric manifestation (such as sleep disturbances, depression, emotional instability and anxiety). On histopathology the finding is similar to lipoma.

Treatment: There are various method of treatment. Liposuction is method of management that is relatively commonly reported in the literature. In Juxta articular form, lipectomy or dermolipectomy has been described as method of amelioration of disease. Pharmacological management mainly targets on analgesics especially non-steroidal anti-inflammatory drugs. Lidocaine can also be used either as intralesional injection, transdermal application or intravenous infusions. There are single reports on beneficial effect of corticosteroids, interferon α-2b, pregabalin, metformin, calcium-channel modulator and infliximab with methotrexate. Recently, deoxycholic acid has also been used for its treatment.

2.4.3 Granular Parakeratosis

Clinical features—It is a rare benign idiopathic reaction pattern. It presents as asymptomatic to pruritic, scaly to hyperkeratotic, red to brown papules and plaques, usually present in the intertriginous area especially axillae. It has been reported with all age group and is more common among women [19].

Pathogenesis—Some authors thought it to be associated with obesity due to its predilection for intertriginous and occluded body surface area. There are two theories underlying its pathogenesis, which includes physical irritation or contact allergy and acquired disorder of cornification. This allergic reaction may be due to deodorants and antiperspirants, which hinder the breakdown of profilaggrin to filaggrin during epidermal differentiation. Histopathology reveal a thickened stratum corneum with abnormal retention of keratohyalin granules as well as intact stratum granulosum.

Treatment—Multiple treatment has been tried with inconsistent result. Topical steroid is the first line of management. Topical steroids alleviate the pruritus but the lesions don't get resolve completely. One case report has also used tretinoin 0.025% for 5 days with complete resolution and another case report showed complete resolution with topical calcitriol ointment for 10 days. There is one another case report, that showed complete resolution with oral isotretinoin. In another case report, complete resolution was achieved with surgical excision with elective mastopexy.

2.4.4 Obesity Associated Lympedematous Mucinosis (OLAM)

Clinical features—OLAM and pretibial stasis mucinosis are uncommon and newly recognised disorders occurring in obese patients or in venous insufficiency. The clinical features consist of asymptomatic, skin-colored to erythematous yellowish semi-translucent papules and nodules progressing to plaques and arising on the legs being associated with erythema, edema, and lymphostasis on the shins. Rarely, vesicles may appear due to severe lymphedema. Stasis mucinosis may present with blue-violet, smooth, pebbly and partially blanchable nodules and plaques, sometimes painful. Further, there may be overlying telangiectasias on the pretibial area along with signs of chronic venous insufficiency [20].

Pathogenesis—It has not been fully explained. Hypoxia may be the prime factor. Obesity leads to lymphatic stasis, which caused local hypoxia with consequent increase in mucin production from fibroblasts. Defect in lymphatic drainage and venous insufficiency leads to interstitial deposition of plasmatic protein, such as fibrinogen, albumin and coagulation factors. This worsens edema decreasing local oxygen delivery and stimulate fibroblasts to further synthesize and deposit glycosaminoglycans.

Treatment—It has a benign course and cause only cosmetic disfigurement. Weight reduction is the mainstay of treatment. Pressure bandage with gradual compression has been found to be useful for venous insufficiency and lymphostasis. Surgical treatment can be considered when there is severe vascular insufficiency.

2.5 Inflammatory Skin Diseases Associated with Obesity

2.5.1 Hidradenitis Suppurativa (HS)

It is an inflammatory, is a chronic recurrent scarring disease of the hair follicle, that usually affect the apocrine gland-bearing areas. Its presentation as deep seated, painful nodules, abscesses, sinus formation, and further leads to scarring. It commonly affects inguinal, axilla ad anogenital region. The exact pathophysiology is still poorly understood. The major comorbid disorders like obesity and smoking are associated with the occurrence or the aggravation of the disease. Obesity plays a pivotal role in HS development supported by increases lesional biomarkers such as IL-17R and S100A8.

Obesity in HS patients increases mechanical friction at flexural sites, further causing injury to follicular opening, occlusion of intrafollicular keratin hydration resulting in narrowing of follicular outlet and elevated levels of pro-inflammatory cytokines results in sweat retention and cause further skin irritation. Obese patients also have increase androgen levels, which further accentuate follicular plugging and deteriorate HS presentation [21].

2.5.2 Psoriasis

Psoriasis has been associated with obesity and metabolic disorders, which includes dyslipidemia, diabetes and non-alcoholic fatty liver disease. IL-17A is a crucial element in the association between obesity and psoriasis. Recent studies found that obesity induces T helper 17 cells, which further secrete IL-17A. Overexpression of IL-17A results in epidermal hyperplasia and strong inflammation, subsequently leads to skin plaques and systemic inflammatory response seen in psoriasis [22]. Proinflammatory mediators get circulated systemically, and induce endothelial dysfunction, hypercoagulation, increase oxidative stress and insulin resistance.

Psoriatic patients with higher BMI have poor respond to systemic therapy and biologics, which are common treatment approaches for this condition. This phenomenon highlights the need for personalized treatment strategies that take into account the patient's BMI and metabolic status. Further, severity of psoriasis decreases with weight loss.

2.5.3 Rosacea

Rosacea can be linked to obesity, but their association is not proved till now. There are few epidemiological studies, which found that patient with high BMI has significantly associated with increased risk of rosacea. Authors also showed positive association between hip and waist circumference and development of rosacea [23].

2.5.4 Hair and Scalp

According to few studies, increase body weight may be associated with premature hair greying (i.e., greying before 30 years of age). An increase in androgen production can be caused by obesity, which can lead to hirsutism. Recently, a study by Papafotiou et al. showed that obese prepubertal girls have higher scalp hair cortisol levels [24]. Cutis verticis gyrata is also associated with insulin resistance, which is one of the prime features of obesity.

2.5.5 *Acne*

Obesity is also associated with Polycystic ovary syndrome, which may cause menstrual irregularities, acne, acanthosis nigricans, HS, seborrhea, hyperinsulinism and androgenetic alopecia. Studies showing correlation of obesity and acne very few and controversial, but these studies suggest that increased BMI may lead to insulin resistance and early menarche and further increase risk of acne.

2.5.6 *Skin Malignancy*

Correlation of obesity and non-melanoma skin cancer is very controversial. Few studies have found lower incidence of basal cell carcinoma among patients with increase weight and BMI [25, 26]. Whereas few other studies found there is no correlation between basal cell carcinoma and BMI. Similarly, correlation between malignant melanoma and obesity is very controversial. Few studies found increase incidence and few other found no correlation [27].

2.6 Conclusion

Various skin manifestations are associated with obesity and its metabolic comorbidities. Increase in BMI is worldwide major health problem and along with increasing prevalence of obesity, the number of cutaneous conditions are also increasing. Dermatologist must be aware about these cutaneous conditions for its early diagnosis, better management and preclusion of its sequalae.

References

1. González-Muniesa P, Mártinez-González MA, Hu FB, Després JP, Matsuzawa Y, Loos RJF, Moreno LA, Bray GA, Martinez JA. Obesity. Nat Rev Dis Primers. 2017;3:17034. https://doi.org/10.1038/nrdp.2017.34. PMID: 28617414. https://pubmed.ncbi.nlm.nih.gov/28617414/.
2. Darlenski R, Mihaylova V, Handjieva-Darlenska T. The link between obesity and the skin. Front Nutr. 2022;9:855573. https://doi.org/10.3389/FrontNutr.2022.855573. PMID: 35369048. https://pubmed.ncbi.nlm.nih.gov/35369048/.
3. Hirt PA, Castillo DE, Yosipovitch G, Keri JE. Skin changes in the obese patient. J Am Acad Dermatol. 2019;81(5):1037–57. https://doi.org/10.1016/j.jaad.2018.12.070. PMID: 31610857. https://pubmed.ncbi.nlm.nih.gov/31610857/.
4. Guida B, Nino M, Perrino NR, Laccetti R, Trio R, Labella S, Balato N. The impact of obesity on skin disease and epidermal permeability barrier status. J Eur Acad Dermatol Venereol. 2010;24(2):191–5. https://doi.org/10.1111/j.1468-3083.2009.03503.x. PMID: 19929936. https://pubmed.ncbi.nlm.nih.gov/22471938/.

5. Poeggeler B, Schulz C, Pappolla MA, Bodó E, Tiede S, Lehnert H, Paus R. Leptin and the skin: a new frontier. Exp Dermatol. 2010;19(1):12–8. https://doi.org/10.1111/j.1600-0625.2009.00930.x. PMID: 19601981. https://pubmed.ncbi.nlm.nih.gov/19601981/.
6. Semkova K, Gergovska M, Kazandjieva J, Tsankov N. Hyperhidrosis, bromhidrosis, and chromhidrosis: fold (intertriginous) dermatoses. Clin Dermatol. 2015;33(4):483–91. https://doi.org/10.1016/j.clindermatol.2015.04.013. ISSN 0738-081X. https://www.sciencedirect.com/science/article/pii/S0738081X15000772.
7. Choonhakarn C, Chaowattanapanit S, Julanon N. Lipodermatosclerosis: a clinicopathologic correlation. Int J Dermatol. 2016;55(3):303–8. https://doi.org/10.1111/ijd.12856. Epub 2015 Aug 14. PMID: 26275890. https://pubmed.ncbi.nlm.nih.gov/26275890/.
8. Das A, Datta D, Kassir M, Wollina U, Galadari H, Lotti T, Jafferany M, Grabbe S, Goldust M. Acanthosis nigricans: a review. J Cosmet Dermatol. 2020;19(8):1857–65. https://doi.org/10.1111/jocd.13544. PMID: 32516476. https://pubmed.ncbi.nlm.nih.gov/32516476/.
9. Phiske MM. An approach to acanthosis nigricans. Indian Dermatol Online J. 2014;5(3):239–49. https://doi.org/10.4103/2229-5178.137765. PMID: 25165638; PMCID: PMC4144206. https://www.ncbi.nlm.nih.gov/pmc/articles/PMC4144206/.
10. Thomas M, Khopkar US. Keratosis pilaris revisited: is it more than just a follicular keratosis? Int J Trichology. 2012;4(4):255–8. https://doi.org/10.4103/0974-7753.111215. PMID: 23766609; PMCID: PMC3681106. https://www.ncbi.nlm.nih.gov/pmc/articles/PMC3681106/.
11. Gerbig AW. Treating keratosis pilaris. J Am Acad Dermatol. 2002;47(3):457. https://doi.org/10.1067/mjd.2002.122733. PMID: 12196765. https://www.jaad.org/article/S0190-9622(02)70065-0/fulltext.
12. Kochet K, Lytus I, Svistunov I, Sulaieva O. [Skin pathology in diabetes mellitus: clinical and pathophysiological correlations (review)]. Georgian Med News. 2017;(273):41–6. Russian. PMID: 29328028. https://pubmed.ncbi.nlm.nih.gov/29328028/.
13. Pandey A, Sonthalia S. Skin tags. [Updated 2022 Aug 1]. In: StatPearls [Internet]. Treasure Island: StatPearls Publishing; 2023. https://www.ncbi.nlm.nih.gov/books/NBK547724/.
14. Lokhande AJ, Mysore V. Striae distensae treatment review and update. Indian Dermatol Online J. 2019;10(4):380–95. https://doi.org/10.4103/idoj.IDOJ_336_18. PMID: 31334056; PMCID: PMC6615396. https://www.ncbi.nlm.nih.gov/pmc/articles/PMC6615396/.
15. Arora G, Patil A, Hooshanginezhad Z, Fritz K, Salavastru C, Kassir M, Goldman MP, Gold MH, Adatto M, Grabbe S, Goldust M. Cellulite: presentation and management. J Cosmet Dermatol. 2022;21:1393–401. https://pubmed.ncbi.nlm.nih.gov/35104044/.
16. Darlenski R, Mihaylova V, Handjieva-Darlenska T. The link between obesity and the skin. Front Nutr. 2022;9:855573. https://doi.org/10.3389/fnut.2022.855573. PMID: 35369048; PMCID: PMC8965625. https://pubmed.ncbi.nlm.nih.gov/35369048/.
17. Shimizu S, Shimizu T, Tateishi Y, Shimizu H. Keratosis follicularis squamosa (Dohi): a follicular keratotic disorder well known in Japan. Br J Dermatol. 2001;144(5):1070–2. https://doi.org/10.1046/j.1365-2133.2001.04202.x. PMID: 11359401. https://pubmed.ncbi.nlm.nih.gov/11359401/.
18. Kucharz EJ, Kopeć-Mędrek M, Kramza J, Chrzanowska M, Kotyla P. Dercum's disease (adiposis dolorosa): a review of clinical presentation and management. Reumatologia. 2019;57(5):281–7. https://doi.org/10.5114/reum.2019.89521. https://www.ncbi.nlm.nih.gov/pmc/articles/PMC6911249/.
19. Ding CY, Liu H, Khachemoune A. Granular parakeratosis: a comprehensive review and a critical reappraisal. Am J Clin Dermatol. 2015;16(6):495–500. https://doi.org/10.1007/s40257-015-0148-2. PMID: 26242230. https://pubmed.ncbi.nlm.nih.gov/26242230/.
20. Ferreli C, Atzori L, Rongioletti F. Obesity-associated lymphedematous mucinosis and stasis mucinosis. Clin Dermatol. 2021;39(2):229–32. https://doi.org/10.1016/j.clindermatol.2020.10.014. Epub 2020 Oct 16. PMID: 34272015. https://pubmed.ncbi.nlm.nih.gov/34272015/.
21. Kaleta KP, Nikolakis G, Hossini AM, Balthasar O, Almansouri D, Vaiopoulos A, Knolle J, Boguslawska A, Wojas-Pelc A, Zouboulis CC. Metabolic disorders/obesity is a primary risk

factor in hidradenitis suppurativa: an immunohistochemical real-world approach. Dermatology. 2022;238(2):251–9. https://doi.org/10.1159/000517017. Epub 2021 Jul 22. PMID: 34293747. https://pubmed.ncbi.nlm.nih.gov/34293747/.

22. Xu C, Ji J, Su T, Wang H-W, Su Z-L. The association of psoriasis and obesity: focusing on IL-17A-related immunological mechanisms. Int J Dermatol Venereol. 2021;4(2):116–21. https://journals.lww.com/ijdv/pages/articleviewer.aspx?year=2021&issue=06000&article=00011&type=Fulltext.
23. Li S, Cho E, Drucker AM, Qureshi AA, Li WQ. Obesity and risk for incident rosacea in US women. J Am Acad Dermatol. 2017;77(6):1083–1087.e5. https://doi.org/10.1016/j.jaad.2017.08.032. Epub 2017 Oct 21. PMID: 29033249. https://pubmed.ncbi.nlm.nih.gov/29033249/.
24. Papafotiou C, Christaki E, van den Akker EL, Wester VL, Apostolakou F, Papassotiriou I, Chrousos GP, Pervanidou P. Hair cortisol concentrations exhibit a positive association with salivary cortisol profiles and are increased in obese prepubertal girls. Stress. 2017;20(2):217–22. Epub 2017. PMID: 28270027. https://pubmed.ncbi.nlm.nih.gov/28270027/.
25. Pelucchi C, Naldi L, Di Landro A, La Vecchia C, Oncology Study Group of Italian Group for Epidemiologic Research in Dermatology. Anthropometric measures, medical history and risk of basal cell carcinoma in an Italian case-control study. Dermatology. 2008;216(3):271–6. https://pubmed.ncbi.nlm.nih.gov/18196938/.
26. Pothiawala S, Qureshi AA, Li Y, Han J. Obesity and the incidence of skin cancer in US Caucasians. Cancer Causes Control. 2012;23(5):717–26. PMID: 22450736. https://www.ncbi.nlm.nih.gov/pmc/articles/PMC3704194/.
27. Sergentanis TN, Antoniadis AG, Gogas HJ, et al. Obesity and risk of malignant melanoma: a meta-analysis of cohort and case-control studies. Eur J Cancer. 2013;49(3):642–57. https://pubmed.ncbi.nlm.nih.gov/23200191/.

Chapter 3
Vitamin D and Skin

Anant Patil and Ramanjit Singh

3.1 Introduction

Skin and its associated structures together help in protection of internal body organs against, harmful effects of external environment. Epidermis, the outer layer acts as a protective barrier against harmful substances. Disturbed functions of skin result in different diseases which lead to adverse impact on physical as well as psychological state of patients. Some systemic diseases including autoimmune disease also have skin manifestations. Thus, condition of skin can reflect not only its status but also pathological changes in the internal organs [1]. Dermatologists are always in search of effective and well tolerated therapies for addressing concerns related to skin disorders or skin manifestations of other systemic disorders.

3.2 Vitamin D and Its Synthesis

Vitamin D is a fat-soluble vitamin, also termed as hormone plays a crucial role in skeletal disorders by regulating calcium and phosphorus levels [1, 2]. It promotes absorption of these minerals [3]. Deficiency of vitamin D is known to cause rickets in children and osteopenia and higher risk of bone fractures in adult population [4].

In humans, synthesis of vitamin D is initiated in the skin from 7-dehydrocholesterol after exposure to sun i.e. ultraviolet B (UVB) radiation [1]. Subsequently after two hydroxylation steps, it is converted to active form, 1,25-dihydroxyvitamin D

A. Patil
Department of Pharmacology, Dr. DY Patil Medical College, Navi Mumbai, India

R. Singh (✉)
Medanta Hospital, Gurgaon, India

R. Singh, N. Sharma (eds.), *A Guide to Hormonal Dermatology*,
https://doi.org/10.1007/978-981-99-7715-4_3

($1,25(OH)_2D$) [5]. First, vitamin D is converted by the liver to 25-hydroxyvitamin D. This is a major circulating form of vitamin D and considered to the best indicator of vitamin D nutritional status. Its levels can be easily estimated. Second hydroxylation occurs in the kidney under the influence of parathyroid hormone. In this step, 25-hydroxyvitamin D is converted to ($1,25(OH)_2D$), the biologically active hormonal form [6]. It is first converted to pre-vitamin D3 (25 OH, Vitamin D3) and finally to vitamin D3 [$1,25(OH)_2$ vitamin D3] after hydroxylation in liver and kidney respectively [4]. Vitamin D is derived from two important sources; sun exposure and diet. Skin exposure to sunlight represents the major source of vitamin D [3]. Vitamin D is available in two distinct forms; vitamin D2 (ergocalciferol) found in yeasts and plants and vitamin D3 (cholecalciferol) with natural dietary sources from salmon, sardines, cod liver oil, shiitake mushrooms, and egg yolk [3].

3.3 Functions of Vitamin D

In addition to this, it plays a role in diversified systemic (extra-skeletal) disorders including those related to heart, central nervous system, reproductive system, infectious diseases, autoimmune conditions, diabetes and cancers [2, 7] by influencing cellular functions [3]. It has been implicated in the increased risk of cardiovascular diseases, certain cancers, autoimmune diseases and infections [4, 8]. Recently, vitamin D has been in discussion due to anti-oxidative, anti-inflammatory and immune response in Coronavirus Disease (COVID-19) [9]. A case control study from India showed strong association of vitamin D status with clinical severity of COVID-19 [10]. Vitamin D is also involved in maintaining skin health and hence, disturbances in its level may contribute to development or progression of different dermatological conditions [2].

3.4 Vitamin D Deficiency

Vitamin D deficiency [25(OH)D level less than 20 ng/mL] is a common concern not only in India but also across the world [11]. It is estimated that more than 50% of the global population is at risk for vitamin D deficiency [4]. Vitamin D deficiency is seen in Indian population of all age groups and both genders. Despite presence of sunshine, prevalence of vitamin D insufficiency or deficiency is common in India [12]. The prevalence of vitamin D deficiency ranges from 40% to 99% [13]. Subclinical vitamin D deficiency is very common in urban as well as rural settings, and across all socioeconomic groups and geographic areas [7]. A study among adults residing in rural West Bengal revealed vitamin D deficiency/insufficiency

Table 3.1 Factors linked to the vitamin D status

• Diet
• Gender
• Body mass index
• Diet
• Socio-economic status
• Aging
• Sun exposure
• Time of the day
• Photoprotection (e.g. sunscreen use)
• Fitzpatrick skin type i.e. skin pigment season
• Latitude
• Physical work/activities
• Alcohol
• Vitamin D receptor polymorphism
• Skin disorders (e.g. photosensitive conditions)

among 67.5% participants [14]. An Indian study reported vitamin D deficiency among 23.46% adolescent children [15]. In another study involving children from Kerala the prevalence of vitamin D deficiency was 11.1%. Protective factors i.e. natural fish diet and the latitude are suggested to be protective factors against deficiency [16]. Girls are reported to be at higher risk for vitamin D deficiency as compared to boys [17]. Causes of vitamin D deficiency may be related inadequate intake, lifestyle, geographical locations or misconception among people that healthy diet contains an adequate vitamin D [4]. Several factors are linked to the status of vitamin D (Table 3.1) [2, 4, 15, 18].

3.5 Skin and Vitamin D

Functions of skin are very closely linked to synthesis and actions of vitamin D [1].

Keratinocytes provide the primary source of vitamin D. On the other hand, vitamin D regulates proliferation and differentiation of keratinocytes. Vitamin D helps as a defense against opportunistic infections [3]. Various cells in the skin express the vitamin D receptor. Moreover, many cell types can convert circulating 25-OH vitamin D to 1,25$(OH)_2$ vitamin D for local use. Considering the mechanisms vitamin D and its analogues have potential for use in psoriasis and other skin diseases [6].

Over the years, there has been increasing interest in vitamin D and its role in skin diseases as seen with increasing number of publications on this topic [19]. Functions of skin regulated by vitamin D are listed in Table 3.2 [20–23].

Table 3.2 Skin functions regulated by vitamin D

• Cellular (keratocyte) proliferation
• Cellular (keratocyte) differentiation
• Apoptosis
• Skin barrier (permeability)
• Innate and adaptive immunity
• Hair follicle cycle
• Tumor formation

3.6 Mechanism of Action of Vitamin D

Biologically active form of vitamin D i.e. 1,25$(OH)_2$D acts by binding to nuclear vitamin D receptors and regulating gene transcription. In some cases, active form of vitamin D exerts its function without regulating gene expression or protein synthesis [21].

Vitamin D level need to be maintained in several skin diseases including atopic dermatitis, psoriasis, acne, vitiligo, lupus erythematosus, polymorphous light eruption, hidradenitis suppurativa, mycosis fungoides, alopecia areata, ichthyosis, androgenic alopecia, melanoma and non-melanoma skin cancer [2, 3, 19].

3.7 Atopic Dermatitis

Atopic dermatitis is an inflammatory skin condition with multiple pathogenic mechanisms including skin barrier impairment and immunological imbalance. Considering immunomodulatory properties, ability to improve cutaneous barrier, role in keratinocyte differentiation, stimulation of filaggrin synthesis and enhancement of expression of antibacterial peptides vitamin D is postulated to have a role in management of atopic dermatitis [3]. A study reported significantly lower median 25(OH)D serum level in patients with atopic dermatitis as compared to healthy controls. There was no significant correlation between vitamin D levels and clinical activity, suggesting its more relation with the level of inflammation than with clinical activity [24]. A meta-analysis of observational studies and randomized controlled trials also reported lower level of vitamin D in patients with all ages with atopic dermatitis and more in children with atopic dermatitis as compared with healthy controls. There was improvement in the clinical scores Scoring Atopic Dermatitis (***SCORAD***) index and Eczema Area and Severity Index (EASI) score after vitamin D supplementation [25]. Another literature review suggested that deficiency of vitamin D is associated with the risk atopic dermatitis and vitamin D may be beneficial in this inflammatory skin condition [20].

3.8 Psoriasis

Due to its chronic nature and frequent relapses, psoriasis is often difficult to treat. Significantly lower median 25(OH)D serum levels are reported in patients with psoriasis than healthy controls. Similar to atopic dermatitis, in patients with psoriasis also, there was no significant correlation between vitamin D levels and clinical activity [24].

A meta-analysis reported significantly low levels of circulating 25[OH]D levels in psoriasis as compared to healthy controls. There is small but statistically significant negative correlation between this level and severity of psoriasis [26]. Similarly, a study showed association between VDR promoter A-1012G polymorphism and risk of psoriasis has also been suggested [27]. However, a meta-analysis reported no genetic variant among the studied to have robust and reproducible association with risk for psoriasis [28]. Vitamin D analogs have a favorable safety profile, and are effective in psoriasis. Topical vitamin D acts by VDR mediated inhibition of epidermal proliferation and inducing keratinocyte differentiation Alteration of antimicrobial peptide expression and reduction in proinflammatory cytokines in psoriasis are the postulated beneficial mechanisms of vitamin D [3].

Oral 1,25$(OH)_2$D (Calcitriol) showed improvement in 88% of 85 patients with psoriasis; whereby 26.5%, 36.2% and 25.3% patients had complete, moderate and slight improvement respectively [29]. Combination of oral calcitriol with acitretin resulted in faster reduction of severity of chronic plaque psoriasis [30]. A open label study reported that twice daily 3 μg/g calcitriol ointment application up to 78 weeks is effective and well-tolerated by patients with chronic plaque psoriasis [31]. Another literature review suggested that deficiency of vitamin D is associated with the risk of psoriasis and vitamin D may be beneficial in the management of psoriasis [20].

3.9 Vitiligo

This is an acquired autoimmune disorder associated with destruction of melanocytes. Vitiligo is associated with reduced levels of serum vitamin D. A meta-analysis of observational studies reported significantly lower levels of serum 25[OH]D in vitiligo as compared to their healthy controls [32]. Association between VDR polymorphisms and 25[OH]D levels is also reported in patients with vitiligo [33]. According to a meta-analysis, there is association of ApaI a allele or BsmI bb genotype with the risk of vitiligo in East Asians [34]. There is no strong evidence for efficacy of oral vitamin D in treatment of vitiligo. In a small study, prolonged vitamin D3 35,000 IU per day for 6 months in patients with psoriasis and vitiligo. Fourteen of 16 patients with vitiligo showed repigmentation in the range of 25–75% [35].

3.10 Skin Cancers

Exposure to sunlight, a source needed the formation of vitamin D can also cause skin cancer, including non-melanocytic cutaneous cancers as well as melanoma [1, 36]. There is conflicting evidence for role of vitamin D and skin cancer risk. A case control study suggested a role for VDR polymorphisms (*BsmI* and *ApaI*) with development of non-melanoma skin cancer. Age of 70 years or younger was a protective against skin cancers. Female and 70 years old or younger were at lower risk of basal cell carcinoma [36]. A meta-analysis of 10 studies involving 6805 skin cancer patients suggested possible significant role of vitamin D receptor FokI and BsmI polymorphism in the risk of cutaneous malignant melanoma and non-melanoma skin cancer. This meta-analysis did not show clear association with vitamin D intake. Further research is necessary to support or clarify the role of diet in these cancers [37]. According to the results of another meta-analysis, circulating level of 25(OH)D is associated with higher risks of melanoma and keratinocyte cancer. It is most likely confounded by sun exposure. There was no association between vitamin D intake skin cancers, except positive associations with risk of basal cell carcinoma [38]. According to a recently published small prospective observational case control study, lower levels of vitamin D may be related to a reduced rate of non-melanoma skin cancer [39].

3.11 Skin Pigmentation

Exposure to ultraviolet radiation stimulates vitamin D synthesis but degrades 5-methyltetrahydrofolate (5-MTHF), the bioactive metabolite of folate. Prevalence of vitamin D deficiency is most common in darkly pigmented people residing in areas with relatively low exposure to ultraviolet radiation. On the contrary, negative relation exists between accumulated ultraviolet exposure and serum folate concentration in people with light pigmented skin [40].

3.12 Anti-aging

Vitamin D_3 is an effective skin protective agent to prevent photoaging. An animal model study showed that liposomes can improve the stability of vitamin D_3 [41]. Antiaging and photoprotective effects are postulated due to immunomodulation, anti-inflammatory actions, regulation of keratinocytes proliferation, epidermal barrier and antioxidative responses [42]. More research is essential to show its beneficial effects as anti-aging substance in human beings. Food fortification with vitamin

D can be an effective option to improve levels of vitamin D and achieve vitamin D sufficiency in the population [7]. In people with deficiency, vitamin D supplements are necessary.

3.13 Other Skin Conditions

Vitamin D deficiency is reported in patients with acne [43], cutaneous lupus erythematosus [44], systemic sclerosis [45], alopecia areata [46], mycosis fungoides [47], and inherited ichtyoses [48]. A small study suggested potential benefit of topical 1,25$(OH)_2D_3$ analogues as prophylactic treatment for polymorphic light eruption [49]. Vitamin D has also been suggested to have a role as adjuvant therapy in patients receiving long-term treatment corticosteroids [19].

3.14 Vitamin D Dosing, Toxicity and Management

Recommended amount of daily intake of vitamin D depends on the age of the person. In adults from 19 to 70 years of age and children from 1 to 13 years of age, 600 IU per day intake is recommended. Adults 71 years and older need 800 IU per day. In children below 1 year of age, 400 IU per day is recommended [50].

For healthy adults, tolerable upper intake level for vitamin D is 4000 IU daily [3]. In patients with signs of vitamin D overdose, supplementation should be discontinued or at least halved and if required, serum calcium levels should be estimated. Toxicity of vitamin D results in hypercalcemia. If the patient has developed intoxication, vitamin D supplementation should be discontinued and the treatment of hypercalcemia should be initiated [51].

3.15 Conclusion

Activities and functions of vitamin D are inseparable from skin. Vitamin D because of its actions on cellular proliferation and differentiation, skin barrier functions, and immune modulation has been studied in many skin disorders. Vitamin D deficiency is seen several skin disorders including atopic dermatitis, psoriasis, vitiligo, polymorphous light eruption, mycosis fungoides, alopecia areata, lupus erythematosus, and melanoma. Mounting evidence is suggesting the role of vitamin D in these skin conditions. More research is required for understanding its exact dose, duration and route of administration.

References

1. Piotrowska A, Wierzbicka J, Zmijewski MA. Vitamin D in the skin physiology and pathology. Acta Biochim Pol. 2016;63:17–29.
2. Kechichian E, Ezzedine K. Vitamin D and the skin: an update for dermatologists. Am J Clin Dermatol. 2018;19:223–35.
3. Bergqvist C, Ezzedine K. Vitamin D and the skin: what should a dermatologist know? G Ital Dermatol Venereol. 2019;154:669–80.
4. Holick MF. Sunlight, UV radiation, vitamin D, and skin cancer: how much sunlight do we need? Adv Exp Med Biol. 2020;1268:19–36.
5. Bikle D, Christakos S. New aspects of vitamin D metabolism and action—addressing the skin as source and target. Nat Rev Endocrinol. 2020;16:234–52.
6. Shahriari M, Kerr PE, Slade K, Grant-Kels JE. Vitamin D and the skin. Clin Dermatol. 2010;28:663–8.
7. Ritu G, Gupta A. Vitamin D deficiency in India: prevalence, causalities and interventions. Nutrients. 2014;6:729–75.
8. Targher G, Pichiri I, Lippi G, Vitamin D. Thrombosis, and hemostasis: more than skin deep. Semin Thromb Hemost. 2012;38:114–24.
9. Slominski RM, Stefan J, Athar M, Holick MF, Jetten AM, Raman C, et al. COVID-19 and vitamin D: a lesson from the skin. Exp Dermatol. 2020;29:885–90.
10. Nimavat N, Singh S, Singh P, Singh SK, Sinha N. Vitamin D deficiency and COVID-19: a case-control study at a tertiary care hospital in India. Ann Med Surg (Lond). 2021;68:102661.
11. Holick MF, Chen TC, Lu Z, Sauter E. Vitamin D and skin physiology: a D-lightful story. J Bone Miner Res. 2007;22(Suppl 2):V28–33.
12. Jan Y, Malik M, Yassen M, Ahmad S, Imran M, Rasool S, et al. Vitamin D fortification of foods in India: present and past scenario. J Steroid Biochem Mol Biol. 2019;193:105417.
13. Aparna P, Muthathal S, Nongkynrih B, Gupta SK. Vitamin D deficiency in India. J Family Med Prim Care. 2018;7:324–30.
14. Garg S, Dasgupta A, Maharana SP, Paul B, Bandyopadhyay L, Bhattacharya A. Sun exposure and vitamin D in rural India: a cross-sectional study. Indian J Public Health. 2018;62:175–81.
15. Chakrabarty S. Prevalence and covariates of vitamin D deficiencies (VDD) among adolescents in India. Indian J Pediatr. 2021;89:751–8. https://doi.org/10.1007/s12098-021-04007-w.
16. Vijayakumar M, Bhatia V, George B. Vitamin D status of children in Kerala, southern India. Public Health Nutr. 2020;23:1179–83.
17. Joshi K, Bhowmik E, Singh N, Bhatia V. Vitamin D status of school-age children in North India. Indian J Pediatr. 2022;89:71–3.
18. Harinarayan CV, Holick MF, Prasad UV, Vani PS, Himbindu G. Vitamin D status and sun exposure in India. Dermatoendocrinology. 2013;5:130–41.
19. Navarro-Trivino FJ, Arias-Santiago S, Gilaberte-Calzada Y. Vitamin D and the skin: a review for dermatologists. Actas Dermosifiliogr (Engl Ed). 2019;110:262–72.
20. Umar M, Sastry KS, Al Ali F, Al-Khylaifi M, Wang E, Chouchane AI. Vitamin D and the pathophysiology of inflammatory skin diseases. Skin Pharmacol Physiol. 2018;31:74–86.
21. Khammissa RAG, Fourie J, Motswaledi MH, Balyaram R, Lemmer J, Feller L. The biological activities of vitamin D and its receptor in relation to calcium and bone homeostasis, cancer, immune and cardiovascular systems, skin biology, and oral health. Biomed Res Int. 2018;2018:9276380.
22. Bikle DD. Vitamin D and the skin. J Bone Miner Metab. 2010;28:117–30.
23. Bikle DD. Vitamin D and the skin: physiology and pathophysiology. Rev Endocr Metab Disord. 2012;13:3–19.
24. Amon U, Baier L, Yaguboglu R, Ennis M, Holick MF, Amon J. Serum 25-hydroxyvitamin D levels in patients with skin diseases including psoriasis, infections, and atopic dermatitis. Dermatoendocrinology. 2018;10:e1442159.

25. Kim MJ, Kim S-N, Lee YW, Choe YB, Ahn KJ. Vitamin D status and efficacy of vitamin D supplementation in atopic dermatitis: a systematic review and meta-analysis. Nutrients. 2016;8:789.
26. Lee YH, Song GG. Association between circulating 25-hydroxyvitamin D levels and psoriasis, and correlation with disease severity: a meta-analysis. Clin Exp Dermatol. 2018;43:529–35.
27. Richetta AG, Silvestri V, Giancristoforo S, Rizzolo P, D'Epiro S, Graziano V, et al. A-1012G promoter polymorphism of vitamin D receptor gene is associated with psoriasis risk and lower allele-specific expression. DNA Cell Biol. 2014;33:102–9.
28. Stefanic M, Rucevic I, Barisic-Drusko V. Meta-analysis of vitamin D receptor polymorphisms and psoriasis risk. Int J Dermatol. 2013;52:705–10.
29. Prez A, Raab R, Chen TC, Turner A, Holick MF. Safety and efficacy of oral calcitriol (1,25-dihydroxyvitamin D3) for the treatment of psoriasis. Br J Dermatol. 1996;134:1070–8.
30. Ezquerra GM, Regaña MS, Millet PU. Combination of acitretin and oral calcitriol for treatment of plaque-type psoriasis. Acta Derm Venereol. 2007;87:449–50.
31. Langner A, Ashton P, Van De Kerkhof PC, Verjans H. A long-term multicentre assessment of the safety and tolerability of calcitriol ointment in the treatment of chronic plaque psoriasis. Br J Dermatol. 1996;135:385–9.
32. Upala S, Sanguankeo A. Low 25-hydroxyvitamin D levels are associated with vitiligo: a systematic review and meta-analysis. Photodermatol Photoimmunol Photomed. 2016;32:181–90.
33. Li K, Shi Q, Yang L, Li X, Liu L, Wang L, et al. The association of vitamin D receptor gene polymorphisms and serum 25-hydroxyvitamin D levels with generalized vitiligo. Br J Dermatol. 2012;167:815–21.
34. Li L, Wu Y, Li L, Cai YF, Geng L, Gao XH, et al. Association of ApaI and BsmI polymorphisms with vitiligo risk: a meta-analysis. Clin Exp Dermatol. 2015;40:794–803.
35. Finamor DC, Sinigaglia-Coimbra R, Neves LCM, Gutierrez M, Silva JJ, Torres LD. A pilot study assessing the effect of prolonged administration of high daily doses of vitamin D on the clinical course of vitiligo and psoriasis. Dermatoendocrinology. 2013;5:222–34.
36. Morgado-Aguila C, Gil-Fernandez G, Davila-Villaobos OR, Perez-Rey J, Rey-Sanchez P, Rodriguez-Velasco F. Vitamin D serum levels and non-melanoma skin cancer risk. Peer J. 2021;9:e12234.
37. Gandini S, Raimondi S, Gnagnarella P, Dore J-F, Maisonneuve P, Testori A. Vitamin D and skin cancer: a meta-analysis. Eur J Cancer. 2009;45:634–41.
38. Mahamat-Saleh Y, Aune D, Schlesinger S. 25-Hydroxyvitamin D status, vitamin D intake, and skin cancer risk: a systematic review and dose-response meta-analysis of prospective studies. Sci Rep. 2020;10:13151.
39. Morgado-Aguila C, Rey-Sanchez P, Gil-Fernandez G, Costa-Fernandez MC, Rodriguez-Velasco FJ. Vitamin D receptor polymorphisms and non-melanoma skin cancer risk: a case-control study. J Clin Med. 2020;9:3819.
40. Wolf ST, Kenney WL. Skin pigmentation and vitamin D-folate interactions in vascular function: an update. Curr Opin Clin Nutr Metab Care. 2021;24:528–35.
41. Bi Y, Xia H, Li L, Lee RJ, Xie J, Liu Z, et al. Liposomal vitamin D_3 as an anti-aging agent for the skin. Pharmaceutics. 2019;11:311.
42. Bocheva G, Slominski RM, Slominski A. The impact of vitamin D on skin aging. Int J Mol Sci. 2021;22:9097.
43. Lim S-K, Ha J-M, Lee Y-H, Lee Y, Seo Y-J, Kim C-D, et al. Comparison of vitamin D levels in patients with and without acne: a case-control study combined with a randomized controlled trial. PLoS One. 2016;11:e0161162.
44. Heine G, Lahl A, Muller C, Worm M. Vitamin D deficiency in patients with cutaneous lupus erythematosus is prevalent throughout the year. Br J Dermatol. 2010;163:863–5.
45. Giuggioli D, Colaci M, Cassone G, Fallahi P, Lumetti F, Spinella A, et al. Serum 25-OH vitamin D levels in systemic sclerosis: analysis of 140 patients and review of the literature. Clin Rheumatol. 2017;36:583–90.

46. Gade VK, Mony A, Munisamy M, Chandrashekar L, Rajappa M. An investigation of vitamin D status in alopecia areata. Clin Exp Med. 2018;18:577–84.
47. Incel Uysal P, Alli N, Hayran Y, Candar T. Mycosis fungoides and vitamin D status: analyses of serum 25-hydroxyvitamin D levels and single nucleotide polymorphisms in the vitamin D receptor gene. Acta Dermatovenerol Croat. 2018;26:8–14.
48. Frascari F, Dreyfus I, Rodriguez L, Gennero I, Ezzedine K, Salles JP, et al. Prevalence and risk factors of vitamin D deficiency in inherited ichthyosis: a French prospective observational study performed in a reference center. Orphanet J Rare Dis. 2014;9:12.
49. Gruber-Wackernagel A, Bambach I, Legat FJ, Hofer A, Byrne SN, Quehenberger F, et al. Randomized double-blinded placebo-controlled intra-individual trial on topical treatment with a 1,25-dihydroxyvitamin D3 analogue in polymorphic light eruption. Br J Dermatol. 2011;165:152–63.
50. Vitamin D fat sheet for consumers. National Institute of Health Office of dietary supplements. https://ods.od.nih.gov/pdf/factsheets/VitaminD-Consumer.pdf. Accessed 1 Mar 2022.
51. Bleizgys A. Vitamin D dosing: basic principles and a brief algorithm (2021 update). Nutrients. 2021;13:4415. https://doi.org/10.3390/nu13124415.

Chapter 4
Thyroid Disorders and the Skin

Abhishek De and Shreya Datta

4.1 Introduction

The human skin is a crucial organ that reflects a variety of endocrine diseases as the interactions of the endocrine and integumentary systems are reflected there. Dysregulation of endocrine hormones results in the appearance of clinically significant cutaneous lesions, which can be recognized by clinicians and hence serve as markers of endocrinopathies. To enhance the patient's health and quality of life, it is crucial for healthcare personnel to be aware of these conditions' occurrence and presentation. An imbalance in thyroid hormone levels has been inherently linked to numerous cutaneous manifestations. As these hormones exert significant influence over the skin, hair, and nails, clinicians need to be well-versed in correctly identifying and diagnosing these diseases.

4.2 Thyroid Gland

4.2.1 Anatomy

The thyroid gland, which weighs between 15 and 25 g in adults, has 2 lateral lobes that are connected by an isthmus that is anterior to the trachea. The thyroid lobes are around 4 cm from superior to inferior, 15–20 mm wide, and 20–39 mm thick. The gland doesn't have real lobulations; just a thin fibrous capsule surrounds it. The thyroid's lateral lobes are situated between the carotid sheath and

A. De (✉) · S. Datta
Department of Dermatology, Calcutta National Medical College, Kolkata, India

R. Singh, N. Sharma (eds.), *A Guide to Hormonal Dermatology*,
https://doi.org/10.1007/978-981-99-7715-4_4

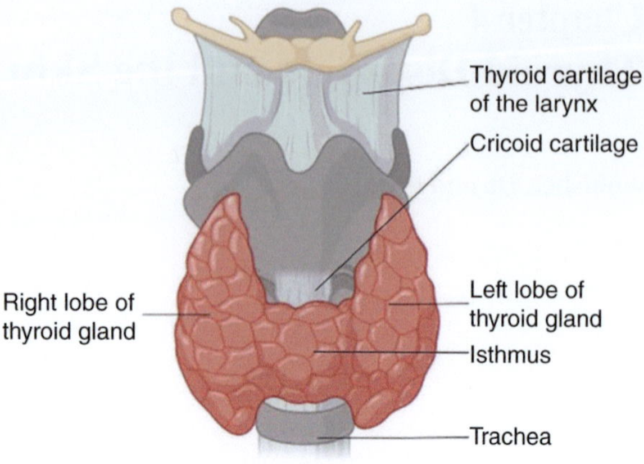

Fig. 4.1 Anatomical structure of the thyroid gland

sternocleidomastoid muscle laterally and the trachea and larynx medially. On the lateral section of the gland, the deep cervical fascia generates a loose false capsule. The superficial fascia and platysma surround the gland on the outside, while the deep cervical fascia condenses on the inside to form the Berry suspensory ligament, which connects the thyroid to the trachea and larynx. The ligament that connects the thyroid to the first two tracheal rings is fastened to the inferior border of the cornu of the cricoid cartilage and reaches inferno-medially onto the tracheal wall. The thyroid is raised during deglutition because of the ligament's connection between it and the trachea. It has been shown that the anterior midline lacks the external thyroid capsule (Fig. 4.1).

4.2.2 Embryology

During the third week of gestation, the thyroid gland begins developing, and it is finished by the 11th week. At the third week of pregnancy, an epithelial growth on the floor of the pharynx directly caudal to the tuberculum impar at the boundary of the first and second pharyngeal pouches indicates the primordium of the medial part of the thyroid gland. By the end of the seventh week of pregnancy, the thyroid will have descended from the floor of the pharynx in front of the hyoid bone and the lingual cartilage to its ultimate position anterior to the trachea. During the fifth week of gestation, the lateral thyroid primordia, which arise from the fourth and fifth pharyngeal pouches and descend to join the medial primordium, have provided up to 30% of the weight of the gland. The parafollicular C cells that make calcitonin are generated by the lateral thyroid anlage, which develops from neural crest cells. The gland has two lateral lobes and a middle isthmus by the by a strip of fibrous or muscular tissue, keeps the thyroid attached to the tongue throughout its migratory journey in-utero (Fig. 4.2).

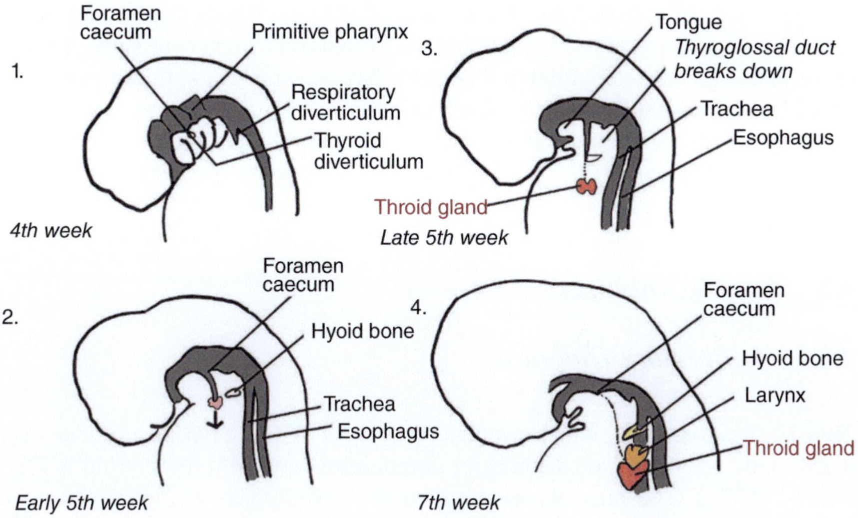

Fig. 4.2 Embryological development of the thyroid gland

4.2.3 Hormones

Thyroid hormones (TH) are potent, naturally occurring, iodinated, amino acid-derived macromolecules. The prohormone L-thyroxine (T4), which is produced exclusively by the thyroid gland's follicular structures, and its major thyromimetically active metabolite T3 (3,3′,5-triiodo-L-thyronine), are referred to as "TH" in most contexts. T3 is produced and released by the thyroid gland in part, although it is mostly created by cellular enzymatic deiodination outside of the thyroid gland. Other TH metabolites (THM) are known to have biological effects in diverse subcellular compartments, which are partly mediated by T3 receptors or other target molecules. T3 is produced and released by the thyroid gland in part, although it is mostly created by cellular enzymatic deiodination outside of the thyroid gland. Other TH metabolites (THM) are known to have biological effects in diverse subcellular compartments, which are partly mediated by T3 receptors or other target molecules [1].

The thyroid hormone receptor mediates direct thyroid hormone action on the skin. Skin tissues have been shown to have all three of the thyroid hormone receptors' well-known binding isoforms. Epidermal homeostasis is significantly regulated by the thyroid hormone. With hypothyroidism, the skin is rough and finely scaled, especially on the extensor extremities. T3 also directly increases the proliferation of both epidermal keratinocytes and dermal fibroblasts, as seen in tissue culture experiments to measure DNA expression [2]. Due to the increased dermal water content and dermal mucopolysaccharides, hypothyroidism often results in pale skin. Inhibiting the formation of hyaluronic acid, fibronectin, and collagen is another impact of thyroid hormone on cultured skin fibroblasts that has been demonstrated in various studies [3]. Hair that has hypothyroidism may be slow-growing, dry, coarse, and brittle. Parallel to this, nails may become brittle, thicker, and sluggish in development. Clinically, thyrotoxicosis cases often has fine, silky hair. Plummer's nails, which are characterized by a concave shape and distal onycholysis, are also visualized.

4.3 Thyroid Diseases

4.3.1 Laboratory Diagnosis

Thyroid function tests, which evaluate the levels of free thyroid hormones and thyrotropin, are the major method for determining how well the thyroid is functioning (TFTs). The majority of the time, these hormones are identified using immunochemical techniques that include an antigen-antibody interaction. According to the test's underlying premise, the immunochemical procedures may be split into two categories: competitive and non-competitive. A manufactured, tagged antigen and an antigen that is already present in a patient's plasma compete for a finite number of antibody binding sites in the competitive technique. The quantity of the "labelled antigen-antibody" combination that is formed is inversely proportional to the analyte's concentration. A laboratory application of a competitive test is the measurement of fT4 and fT3 [4]. Two kinds of antibodies are used in non-competitive binding tests: capture and labelled. The first one, which is typically coated on a solid phase, picks up analyte particles with a particular epitope on their surface. The reaction mixture is then supplemented with a conjugate, which is a suspension of labelled (signal) antibodies. The "sandwich assay," which combines the capture antibody and the antibody that has been labelled with an antigen, is created when these antibodies attach to a different piece of the molecule being evaluated. TSH is measured using a non-competitive assay.

An essential stage in the diagnosis of thyroid problems is now the evaluation of anti-thyroid antibodies. The antibodies that are most often seen in daily life include: TG, anti-TSHR, and anti-TPO.

It is essential to prevent misleading findings brought on by interferences in the lab. Laboratory interference comes in two forms: positive, which causes a falsely increased test result, and negative, which causes a falsely lowered test result. The immunoassay may be impacted by several circumstances at all phases of testing.

The prominent ones include heterophilic antibodies, macro TSH, biotin, anti-streptavidin, anti-ruthenium antibodies, and thyroid hormone autoantibodies.

4.3.2 Types and Epidemiology

Thyroid diseases can broadly be classified as either hypothyroidism or hyperthyroidism. Hypothyroidism is the pathological condition of thyroid hormone deficiency. There are four different forms of hypothyroidism: primary (caused by a lack of thyroid hormone), secondary (by a lack of TSH), tertiary (by a lack of thyrotropin-releasing hormone), and peripheral (by a lack of thyroid hormones outside of the gland, i.e., extra-thyroidal). The most common type of primary hypothyroidism is chronic autoimmune thyroiditis, often known as Hashimoto's disease. Pituitary or hypothalamic dysfunctions brought on by head injuries, Sheehan's syndrome, radiotherapy, surgery, etc. are associated with central hypothyroidism. Rarely occurring peripheral hypothyroidism is brought on by abnormal deiodinase three enzyme expression.

Hyperthyroidism results from an increased availability of thyroid hormone. Some prominent disorders include Graves' disease—an autoimmune disorder resulting in the proliferation of lymphocytes and plasma cells, toxic nodular goiter, T3 thyrotoxicosis, iatrogenic and factitious hyperthyroidism [5].

Hashimoto's disease (AITD) is the most common thyroid disorder accounting for an expected prevalence of about 5% [6]. According to epidemiological research, women are at a larger risk than males. The occurrence of Hashimoto's hypothyroidism varies geographically and is age-related. Compared to the state of iodine deficiency, its occurrence is greater in the former. Furthermore, antithyroid antibody (ATA) frequency varies by race, rises with age, and falls with smoking. Autoimmune skin disorders (AISD) such pemphigus, bullous pemphigoid, vitiligo, and alopecia are greatly influenced by AITD.

4.3.3 Hyperthyroidism

Hyperthyroidism is a state of the thyroid gland where it produces an excess of thyroid hormones, exceeding the body's requirements. This condition of the body has been attributed to a number of factors, including excessive dietary intake of thyroxine or iodine, thyroiditis (including the autoimmune disease Graves' disease), toxic multinodular goiter, a pituitary adenoma that secretes thyrotropin, metastatic follicular cancer of the thyroid gland or molar pregnancy. Almost all of the dermatological signs like pretibial myxedema, along with ophthalmopathy are, however, associated with Grave's disease. The ophthalmologic and dermatologic signs are thought to be autoimmune-mediated rather than connected to the thyroid hormone titer. Hyperthyroidism is reflected through varied dermatological manifestations like warm, moist, and pruritic skin, bearing similarities with infantile skin. T3/T4 is believed to mediate these manifestations directly.

The surge in blood flow brought on by peripheral vasodilation causes the warmth, face flushing, and palmar erythema seen in patients. Furthermore, excessive perspiration is seen, particularly on the patient's palms and soles. There is evident fine, silky scalp hair, which is sometimes accompanied by alopecia. The typical "Plummer's nail," which may also be found in hypothyroidism and psoriasis, is present in 5% of individuals who have nail findings [7]. There have also been reports of hyperpigmentation that follows the same typical distribution as Addison's illness (creases of the palms and soles, gingiva, and buccal mucosa).

Another uncommon condition associated with hypothyroidism is scleromyxedema, which consists of many hard, white, yellow, or pink papules. Weight loss, vascular disease, and myopathy are often present along with it, and it is typically noticeable on the face, trunk, axillae, and limbs. Skin lesions are caused by a buildup of acid mucopolysaccharides, mostly hyaluronic acid, in the dermis together with fibrocystic invasion. It leads to swelling of the digits and sparing of the palms and soles.

Pretibial myxedema is a dermal fibroblastic growth that affects 0.5–4% of patients. It triggers the release of cytokines and local glycosaminoglycans, which leads to mild to moderate skin thickening that can visually range from a "peau d'orange" appearance to extensive infiltrative lesions which coalesce to resemble elephantiasis vurrucosa nostra.

This can occur in other areas of the body (e.g., face, preradial area, scalp, neck, extremities, torso) too. This may also develop in other body parts, such as the face, scalp, neck, limbs, and torso. The early lesions often present as hard, uneven plaques or lumps that range in color from pink to purple brown. The involvement of the hair follicles gives rise to the characteristic dimpled appearance.

Several theories exist which try to explain the pathogenesis of the disease. Thyrotropin (TSH) and TSH receptor antibody binding, in addition to the extracellular domain of the TSH receptor encoded by RNA, were found in pretibial fibroblasts, according to Chang et al.'s research [8]. Thyroid autoantibodies cause fibroblasts to overproduce glycosaminoglycans, which results in their buildup. Another view contends that the pathophysiology of this clinical symptom is really caused by local variables (trauma and edema) in conjunction with asymptomatic connective dysregulation, suggesting that the autoimmune state may not be the only cause of the dermatopathies of Graves' illness [7].

This condition serves to be an extremely difficult one to cure, even if the hyperthyroidism is corrected. Topical triamcinolone has proven to be effective among 150 patients suffering from pretibial myxedema, as reported in this study [9].

Intravenous immunoglobulin, octreotide, and intravenous pulse steroids followed by oral steroids constitute additional treatments. In order to gauge skin thickness and determine the effectiveness of treatment, ultrasonography serves to be a useful diagnostic tool.

4.3.4 Hypothyroidism

Hypothyroidism is primarily described biochemically as a thyroid hormone-deficient disorder. Blatant or clinical primary hypothyroidism is defined as TSH levels beyond the guideline range and free thyroxine levels below the reference range. The requirements for moderate or subclinical hypothyroidism, which is frequently seen as a sign of early thyroid failure, include TSH readings above the reference range and free thyroxine concentrations within the usual limits. Hypothyroidism is more common both in people with a reasonably high iodine consumption and in those that are severely deficient in iodine, depending on iodine status.

One of several clinical features of hypothyroidism is the appearance of dry skin and coarse hair, and thus hypothyroidism can be expressed in the form of several dermatological manifestations such as xeroderma, pilose keratosis, palmoplantar keratoderma, hypohidrosis, generalized myxedema, purpura, ecchymosis, etc. [10].

Epidermal signs play a crucial role as external indicators of thyroid illness. Sebaceous glands, keratinocytes, fibroblasts, and hair follicles all have thyroid hormone receptors. In the skin, thyroid hormone-responsive genes and parts of the hypothalamic-pituitary-thyroid axis were found. In addition to altering the skin barrier, lamellar granule formation, the production of Odland bodies, and the activity of cholesterol sulphate cycle enzymes, hypothyroidism also stimulates the buildup of mucopolysaccharides and water in the dermis.

Patients with hypothyroidism experience a yellowish tone in their skin due to an increase in carotene in the dermis.

Hypohidrosis, or a reduction in sweating and sebum excretion, is a thyroid disorder complication that worsens skin dryness. The cutaneous condition known as mucinosis or generalized myxedema is indicative with hypothyroidism. Patients have widespread edema which is particularly noticeable in the periorbital and acral regions. A universal rise in dermal acid mucopolysaccharides, mainly hyaluronic acid and chondroitin sulphate, is the cause of this illness. Generalized myxedema may sometimes mimic the musculoskeletal signs and symptoms of polymyositis. All these disorders contribute to the development of friction-induced intraepidermal bullae as well as purpura and ecchymosis. In fact, Le Brun et al. [11] recommended thyroid hormone assays in any patient presenting pretibial bullae in their report of a case of hypothyroidism and pretibial epidermolysis bullosa, which rapidly regressed after hormone therapy (Fig. 4.3).

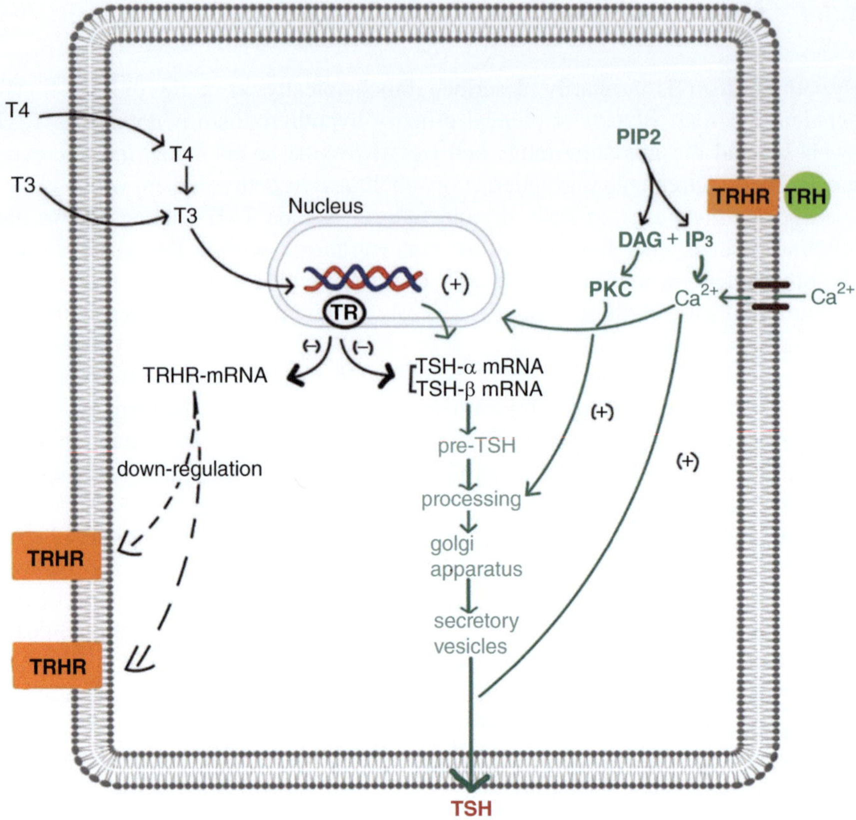

Fig. 4.3 The complex regulatory mechanisms governing the thyroid hormone and TSH levels in our body

4.4 Thyroid Cancer

The most prevalent kind of thyroid cancer is papillary thyroid cancer, which is followed in decreasing order by follicular, medullary, and anaplastic carcinoma [12].

The lymphocytic expansion of the thyroid gland is a side effect of chronic instances of goiter in Hashimoto's thyroiditis. With a 7% frequency of occurrence in the general population, thyroglossal duct cysts—another dermatological presentation of thyroid disease, is the most prevalent representation of midline neck lumps seen in children [13]. They may develop anywhere along the thyroid's embryologic migration path from the tongue base at the foramen cecum to the inferior neck. They are an embryologic residue resulting from an inability to seal the thyroglossal duct.

The most common sign of thyroglossal duct malignancies (TGDCs) is a movable midline neck tumour located close to the hyoid bone.

The initial cutaneous manifestation is a palpable thyroid nodule observed during routine clinical examinations. More advanced stages are characterized by significant distortion of the neck anatomy due to the size of the nodule.

Although rare, cutaneous metastasis from thyroid carcinoma has been reported in 43 situations, based on a review by Dahl et al. [14]. Cutaneous metastases are more commonly observed in follicular carcinoma rather than papillary carcinoma, as reported by Koller et al. Occurring against the backdrop of disseminated neoplastic disease, it was discovered that papillary carcinoma was most commonly implicated in skin metastases, occurring in almost 41% of cases, followed by follicular carcinoma at 28% [15, 16]. Skin metastasis, which can be easily misdiagnosed as a primary adnexal skin tumor, presents as violaceous, or blue-colored nodules slowly growing either as solitary lesions or grouped into multiple, erythematous papules. In the Dahl et al. research [14], over two-thirds of patients indicated that their scalp was most often affected. Given the extensive dermal capillary network that nourishes the scalp and face serving as the ideal conduit for metastatic cells, hence the metastases remain confined to these areas of the upper body.

4.5 Alopecia Areata

Non-scarring hair loss is a hallmark of the condition known as alopecia areata. AA is a hereditary disorder that is influenced by several genetic variables. From 10% to 25% of the time, a positive family history is obvious. In 60% of the patients, which were mostly autoimmune in nature, a connection between diffuse alopecia and thyroid disorders was established. According to recent studies, systemic auto-reactive cells, which are also present in autoimmune hypothyroid disorders, are partly to blame for the typical hair loss in AA [15, 16]. Alopecia areata is believed to be caused by autoimmune processes, according to mounting data. Due to the absence of HLA class I molecule expression under normal circumstances, hair follicles are generally shielded from immunological responses. The invasion of lymphocytes, including T cells and natural killer cells, into the hair follicles, is evident in autoimmune thyroid illness, however. The alopecia areata is exacerbated by this. Patients with autoimmune hyperthyroidism and autoimmune hypothyroidism were shown to have considerably greater rates of alopecia than the control group. The development of alopecia areata is seriously threatened by thyroid autoimmune diseases. All therapies, however, are intended to stop hair loss and encourage regrowth since there is no known cure for the underlying cause of AA. During 1 year of follow-up of AA cases, 34–50% of people see a spontaneous restoration in their hair growth. Up to 20% of patients with the condition will develop alopecia totalis as it progresses over time [17, 18].

4.6 Chronic Idiopathic Urticaria

A pioneering study involving 220 patients suffering from thyroid dysfunction along with 90 healthy individuals as control reported that 56.8% [19] suffered from apparent skin-related pathologies. The fact that diseases like chronic urticaria (6.8%), vitiligo (6.8%), and pruritus were discovered to have a higher rate of occurrence among patients suffering from thyroid diseases as opposed to the control reiterates the relationship between this gland and the normal functioning of the skin.

Several theories have been suggested to explain this common link between AITD and CSU, with the most widely accepted one being the dysregulation of common immunological pathways, an increase in IL-6 levels, a decrease in the count of Treg lymphocytes, and an increase in Th17 lymphocytes [20].

Women with both CU and Hashimoto thyroiditis showed stronger positive results at the Autologous Serum Skin Test (ASST), as well as higher skin TSHR expression, according to a recent research on CU patients with or without Hashimoto thyroiditis [21]. The research found that the TSHR expression was favourably linked with both ASST measures and anti-TPO blood levels. There is a clear manifestation that skin TSHR expression and CU, Hashimoto thyroiditis, and thyroid disease all have a connection [21]. Last but not least, it has been shown that 60% of CU patients had significant levels of IgE-anti-TPO autoantibodies. This indicates that mast cell activation in CU patients may be auto-allergic in origin since it positively linked with the levels of IgG-anti-TPO autoantibodies.

4.7 Other Thyroid Dermopathies

Two major clinical conditions are associated with autoimmune disorders of the thyroid gland, which have a 5% prevalence rate: (a) chronic lymphocytic infiltration that results in Hashimoto's thyroiditis, which causes hypothyroidism, and (b) Graves' disease, which is distinguished by hyperthyroidism [22]. In Hashimoto's thyroiditis, self-reactive CD4+ T lymphocytes stimulate B cells to create anti-Tg and anti-TPO antibodies. Thyrocytes undergo apoptosis when CD8+ T cells are simultaneously activated, gradually causing the gland to fibrose. There is a subsequent decrease in the secretion of thyroid hormones, leading to a state of hypothyroidism. Grave's disease has different pathogenesis where stimulating TSH receptor antibody (immunoglobulin G in nature) binding to the TSH receptor leads to the disruption of the normal negative feedback system and an unopposed systemic action of T3 and T4 [23].

4.8 Dermatitis Herpetiformis

Dermatitis herpetiformis (DH) is an autoimmune dermatological condition characterized by blisters and pruritus due to IgA deposits in perilesional skin [24]. Studies have correlated DH with several other autoimmune pathologies like AITD, mainly Hashimoto's thyroiditis [25]. In fact, according to many studies, between 18% and 48% of DH patients exhibit anti-TPO autoantibodies [25]. Genetic investigations have shown that immune-mediated dysregulation is a frequent precipitator reason in both dermatitis herpetiformis and autoimmune thyroid disease patients, showing an elevated incidence of HLA-B8 and HLA-DRw3 in both illnesses [26].

4.9 Vitiligo

Vitiligo is a distressing dermatopathy characterized by the appearance of well-circumscribed milky cutaneous macules due to the immune-mediated destruction of melanocytes. Histological studies on lesional skin samples have shown dermal inflammation accompanied by the complete or nearly complete absence of melanocytes at stratum basale [27]. With a prevalence of 0.5–1% of the world's population coupled with the obvious disfiguring effects on the skin, the patient's quality of life and mental health is also negatively affected. A recent meta-analysis revealed that in 14.3% of vitiligo patients demonstrated having AITD, with a 20.8% positive reaction to thyroid-specific antibodies (i.e. anti-TPO, anti-Tg, and TRAb) [28].

Thirty-seven susceptibility genes for vitiligo have been identified by candidate gene association studies, genome-wide association studies (GWAS) and genome-wide linkage studies, of which 15 are shared with AITD [29]. Out of these, nine loci are potentially considered to be involved in the pathogenesis of both diseases, out of which organ-specific genes exist coding for TYR, Tg, and TSHR [30]. The study also found that AIS1, an autoimmunity susceptibility locus on chromosome 1 commonly found in both vitiligo and Hashimoto's thyroiditis (HT), has 27 genes mapping to it [30]. All this evidence points toward the fact that AITD and vitiligo have a linked set of susceptibility genes, thus emphasizing the need for screening tests for thyroid diseases in vitiligo patients as an early diagnosis can significantly reduce mortality and improve the patient's QoL.

4.10 Psoriasis

An immune-mediated dermatopathy with a long course, psoriasis is characterized by well-delineated, erythematous plaques that are histologically classified as acanthosis and hyperkeratosis. The relationship between psoriasis and blood levels of free thyroxine (FT4), TSH, and anti-TPO autoantibodies was examined in recent

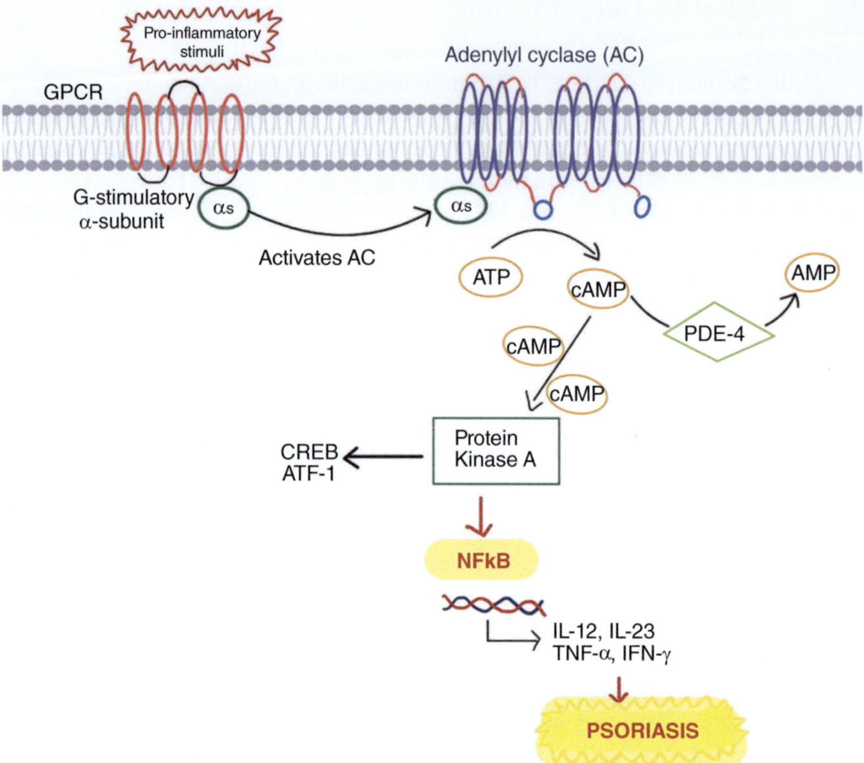

Fig. 4.4 Pathophysiology of psoriasis

research involving 8214 subjects. According to the research, there was a positive, but marginally non-significant, association between the levels of TSH and/or FT4 in the blood [31]. Nevertheless, a substantial correlation between psoriasis and the presence of anti-TPO autoantibodies, as well as hypo- and hyperthyroidism conditions, was found when the aforementioned authors conducted a meta-analysis including four additional published case studies [32] (Fig. 4.4).

The thyroid hormones and their receptors that are produced in the skin are necessary for boosting skin proliferation because they operate as intrinsic regulators of skin irritation. This is most probably the consequence of interference with activator protein 1 (AP-1), nuclear factor kappa-light-chain-enhancer of activated B cells (NF-B), signal transducer and activator of transcription 3 (STAT3) activation, and, most critically, by raising the quantity of epidermal growth factor (promoting keratinocytic differentiation and development). The thyroid hormones T3 and T4 also enhance the Epidermal growth factor (EGF) at the same time, which results in epidermal hyperplasia and psoriasis vulgaris.

4.11 Miscellaneous Diseases

Pemphigus foliaceus and pemphigus vulgaris are a few of the autoimmune diseases occurring simultaneously along with immune-mediated thyroid disease (specifically, Graves' disease) [33]. Case reports of HLA-DR3 and HLA-DR4 among patients with Graves' disease and pemphigus vulgaris have raised speculation regarding the genetic linkage existing between these diseases and AITD. Patients suffering from Hashimoto's thyroiditis and Graves' disease have also been seen to be afflicted by bullous pemphigoid in a few case reports [34]. All these sporadic cases reported in medical literature warrant a detailed investigation analyzing the exact pathophysiological feature linking these diseases together.

The development of thyrocytes and accompanying increased hormone secretion are believed to be triggered by mutations in the G-protein signalling pathway, which are thought to be the second most frequent endocrinopathy linked to McCune Albright Syndrome (MAS). Further contributing to the solitary, segmental appearance of light brown pigmented macules across the posterior neck, sacrum, and neck is the concomitant overactivity of the tyrosinase enzyme.

Despite the fact that there have been a few reports of oral mucosal pigmentation, McCune-Albright syndrome (MAS) is not often considered when determining the cause of oral lentigosity. Oral café au lait pigmentation should be recognised as a clinical sign of MAS, which has related systemic symptoms, since the clinical phenotype of MAS changes owing to mosaicism.

4.12 Conclusion

Several dermatological skin conditions are related to a dysfunction of the thyroid gland like hyperthyroidism, thyroid cancer, hypothyroidism, etc. Abnormal thyroid hormone levels or thyroid autoantibodies may lead to the appearance of these cutaneous signs which act as an important diagnostic tool for healthcare professionals to intervene in a timely manner and preserve the lifespan of the patient.

References

1. Moeller LC, Broecker-Preuss M. Transcriptional regulation by nonclassical action of thyroid hormone. Thyroid Res. 2011;4(Suppl 1):S6.
2. Safer JD, Fraser LM, Ray S, Holick MF. Topical triiodothyronine stimulates epidermal proliferation, dermal thickening, and hair growth in mice and rats. Thyroid. 2001;11:717–24.
3. Smith TJ, Murata Y, Horwitz AL, et al. Regulation of glycosaminoglycan synthesis by thyroid hormone in vitro. J Clin Invest. 1982;70:1066–73.

4. Haddad RA, Giacherio D, Barkan AL. Interpretation of common endocrine laboratory tests: technical pitfalls, their mechanisms and practical considerations. Clin Diabetes Endocrinol. 2019;5:12.
5. Zellmann HE. Hyperthyroidism. Med Clin North Am. 1972;56(3):717–24.
6. Yoo WS, Chung HK. Recent advances in autoimmune thyroid diseases. Endocrinol Metab. 2016;31:379–85.
7. De Bruin TW, Braverman LE, Brown RS. Heterogeneity of TSH receptor-binding antibodies in Hashimoto's thyroiditis and Graves' disease. Am J Med Sci. 1990;299:291–7.
8. Bahn RS. TSH receptor expression in orbital tissue and its role in the pathogenesis of Graves' ophthalmopathy. J Endocrinol Investig. 2004;27:216–20.
9. Di Cerbo A, Di Paola R, Menzaghi C, et al. Graves' immunoglobulins activate phospholipase A2 by recognizing specific epitopes on thyrotropin receptor. J Clin Endocrinol Metab. 1999;84:3283–92.
10. Niepomniszcze H, Huaier Amad R. Skin disorders and thyroid diseases. J Endocrinol Investig. 2001;24(8):628–38. https://doi.org/10.1007/bf03343905.
11. Le Brun V, Boulinguez S, Bouyssou-Gauthier ML, Roux J, Labrousse F, Bonnetblanc JM, Bedane C. Pretibial epidermolysis bullosa and hypothyroidism. Ann Dermatol Venereol. 2000;127:184–7.
12. Ain KB. Management of undifferentiated thyroid cancer. Baillieres Best Pract Res Clin Endocrinol Metab. 2000;14:615–29.
13. Quintanilla-Dieck L, Penn EB. Congenital neck masses. Clin Perinatol. 2018;45(4):769–85.
14. Dahl PR, Brodland DG, Goellner JR, et al. Thyroid carcinoma metastatic to the skin: a cutaneous manifestation of a widely disseminated malignancy. J Am Acad Dermatol. 1997;36:531–7.
15. Koller BA, Tourtelot JB, Pak HS, et al. Papillary and follicular thyroid carcinoma metastatic to the skin: a case report and review of the literature. Thyroid. 1998;8:1045–50.
16. Naik PP, Farrukh SN. Association between alopecia areata and thyroid dysfunction. Postgrad Med. 2021;133(8):895–8.
17. Hammerschmidt M, Mulinari BF. Efficacy and safety of methotrexate in alopecia areata. An Bras Dermatol. 2014;89(5):729–34.
18. O'Donnell BF, Francis DM, Swana GT, Seed PT, Kobza Black A, Greaves MW. Thyroid autoimmunity in chronic urticaria. Br J Dermatol. 2005;153:331–5.
19. Berghi NO. Immunological mechanisms implicated in the pathogenesis of chronic urticaria and Hashimoto thyroiditis. Iran J Allergy Asthma Immunol. 2017;16(4):358–66.
20. Kasperska-Zajac A, Grzanka A, Damasiewicz-Bodzek A. IL-6 transsignaling in patients with chronic spontaneous urticaria. PLoS One. 2015;10:e0145751.
21. Silvares MR, Fortes MR, Nascimento RA, Padovani CR, Miot HA, Nogueira CR, et al. Thyrotropin receptor gene expression in the association between chronic spontaneous urticaria and Hashimoto's thyroiditis. Int J Dermatol. 2017;56:547–52.
22. Muhali F-S, Song R-H, Wang X, Shi X-H, Jiang W-J, Xiao L, et al. Genetic variants of BANK1 gene in autoimmune thyroid diseases: a case-control association study. Exp Clin Endocrinol Diabetes. 2013;121(9):556–60.
23. Nikiforov YE, Biddinger PW, Thompson LDR. Diagnostic pathology and molecular genetics of the thyroid. Philadelphia: Wolters Kluwer—Lippincott Williams & Wilkins; 2009.
24. Ávalos-Díaz E, Herrera ER. Dermatological autoimmune diseases. In: Anaya JM, Shoenfeld Y, Rojas-Villarraga A, Levy RA, Cervera R, editors. Autoimmunity: from bench to bedside. Bogota: El Rosario University Press; 2013. p. 597–610.
25. Zettinig G, Weissel M, Flores J, Dudczak R, Vogelsang H. Dermatitis herpetiformis is associated with atrophic but not with goitrous variant of Hashimoto's thyroiditis. Eur J Clin Investig. 2000;30:53–7.
26. Benvenga S, Guarneri F. Molecular mimicry and autoimmune thyroid disease. Rev Endocr Metab Disord. 2016;17:485–98.
27. Spritz RA. Shared genetic relationships underlying generalized vitiligo and autoimmune thyroid disease. Thyroid. 2010;20:745–54. https://doi.org/10.1089/thy.2010.1643.

28. Vrijman C, Kroon MW, Limpens J, Leeflang MM, Luiten RM, van der Veen JP, et al. The prevalence of thyroid disease in patients with vitiligo: a systematic review. Br J Dermatol. 2012;167:1224–35.
29. Alkhateeb A, Stetler GL, Old W, Talbert J, Uhlhorn C, Taylor M, et al. Mapping of an autoimmunity susceptibility locus (AIS1) to chromosome 1p31.3-p32.2. Hum Mol Genet. 2002;11:661–7. https://doi.org/10.1093/hmg/11.6.661.
30. Kim YC, Kim YJ, Kang HY, Sohn S, Lee ES. Histopathologic features in vitiligo. Am J Dermatopathol. 2008;30:112–6.
31. Khan SR, Bano A, Wakkee M, Korevaar TIM, Franco OH, Nijsten TEC, et al. The association of autoimmune thyroid disease (AITD) with psoriatic disease: a prospective cohort study, systematic review and meta-analysis. Eur J Endocrinol. 2017;177:347–59.
32. Wu JJ, Nguyen TU, Poon KY, Herrinton LJ. The association of psoriasis with autoimmune diseases. J Am Acad Dermatol. 2012;67:924–30.
33. Ljubojevic S, Lipozenčić J. Autoimmune bullous diseases associations. Clin Dermatol. 2012;30:17–33.
34. Collins MT, Singer FR, Eugster E. McCune-Albright syndrome and the extraskeletal manifestations of fibrous dysplasia. Orphanet J Rare Dis. 2012;7(Suppl 1):S4.

Chapter 5
Cutaneous Manifestations of Diabetes

Vineet Relhan and Garima Dabas

5.1 Introduction

Diabetes mellitus (DM) is one of the most important health care challenges around the world and is associated with significant morbidity and mortality. Epidemiological studies have suggested that by 2025, the number of patients with DM will reach 250–300 million globally [1]. DM can affect any organ system in the body including the skin. Cutaneous manifestations of DM are common and have been reported in 30–70% of patients with diabetes [2]. For ease of understanding, in this chapter, we have classified the cutaneous manifestations of diabetes into the following categories (Table 5.1):

1. Cutaneous manifestations associated with complications of diabetes (vascular damage, neurological damage)
2. Cutaneous infections (bacterial, viral, fungal)
3. Dermatologic diseases associated with insulin resistance, obesity and hyperinsulinemia
4. Skin manifestations associated with diabetes
5. Treatment-related skin manifestations

Amongst the above-mentioned manifestations, a few are specific are to diabetes while others can be observed in a plethora of conditions (Tables 5.2 and 5.4). Certain

V. Relhan (✉)
Department of Dermatology, Venereology, and Leprology, Maulana Azad Medical College and Associated Lok Nayak Hospital, New Delhi, India

G. Dabas
Department of Dermatology, Venereology, and Leprology, Maulana Azad Medical College, New Delhi, India

R. Singh, N. Sharma (eds.), *A Guide to Hormonal Dermatology*,
https://doi.org/10.1007/978-981-99-7715-4_5

Table 5.1 Cutaneous manifestations of diabetes at a glance

1. Cutaneous manifestation associated with complications of diabetes
(a) Macroangiopathy—atherosclerosis
(b) Microangiopathy
• Diabetic dermopathy
• Rubeosis faciei
• Palmar erythema
• Periungual telangiectasia
• Diabetic foot syndrome
• Pigmented purpuric dermatosis
(c) Neuropathic—diabetic foot syndrome, neuropathic arthropathy (Charcot's foot)
2. Infectious
(a) Bacterial infections:
• Carbunculosis
• Ecthyma
• Erysipelas
• Folliculitis
• Furunculosis
• Green nail syndrome
• Impetigo
• Malignant external otitis
• Necrotizing fasciitis
(b) Fungal infections:
• Angular cheilitis
• Candidal balanitis
• Candidal paronychia
• Dermatophytosis
• Monilial paronychia
3. Cutaneous manifestations associated with obesity and metabolic syndrome
(a) Acanthosis Nigricans
(b) Eruptive xanthomas
(c) Acrocordon
4. Skin diseases aggravated by diabetes mellitus
(a) Granulomatous disorders
• Necrobiosis lipoidica
• Generalised granuloma annulare
(b) Stiff skin and joints
• Scleroderma-like skin change
• Limited joint mobility
• Scleredema diabeticorum
• Huntley's Papules
(c) Diabetic bullae
(d) Acquired perforating dermatosis
(e) Miscellaneous disorders—Ichthyosis, Xerosis, Pruritus, Keratosis Pilaris, Yellow skin and nails, Psoriasis, Lichen Planus, Vitiligo, Hidradenitis Suppurativa, Glucagonoma

Table 5.1 (continued)

5. Dermatologic complications of diabetes treatment
(a) Insulin—Lipohypertrophy, Lipoatrophy, Allergic reaction
(b) Oral hypoglycemic agent—bullous pemphigoid, SJS, Maculopapular rash

Table 5.2 Dermatologic manifestations of diabetes by category

Specific cutaneous markers	Nonspecific conditions
Diabetic dermopathy	Rubeosis faciei
Diabetic bullae	Palmar erythema
Scleredema diabeticorum	Nailbed erythema
Necrobiosis lipoidica	Pigmented purpuric dermatoses
Generalized granuloma annulare	Acrochordons
	Generalized pruritus
	Thick skin
	Yellow skin and nails

Table 5.3 Most frequent skin disorders among type 1 and type 2 DM

Type 1 diabetes mellitus	Type 2 diabetes mellitus
Necrobiosis lipoidica diabeticorum	Generalized granuloma annulare
Diabetic bullae	Scleredema diabeticorum
Vitiligo vulgaris	Diabetic dermopathy
Periungual telangiaecstasia	Acanthosis nigricans
	Acrochordons
	Psoriasis

cutaneous manifestations are more common in patients with type 1 diabetes as compared to type 2 (Table 5.3). However, often there is no clear distinction between the two types.

5.2 Pathogenesis

Hyperglycemia in DM can arise due to a defect in insulin secretion, insulin action, or both.

It can cause non-enzymatic glycation of proteins, lipids, and nucleic acids, resulting in increased production of advanced glycation end-products (AGEs). These AGEs are responsible for complications associated with diabetes such as microangiopathy, microangiopathy and neuropathy. Diabetic microangiopathy is histologically characterized by the proliferation of endothelial cells, loss of pericytes, and deposition of PAS-positive material on the basement membrane of arterioles, capillaries, and venules [3]. Oxidative stress plays an important role in inducing endothelial lesion, leucocyte adhesion, altered coagulation, and inflammation [3]. Macroangiopathy in diabetic patients leads to endothelial dysfunction, low vessel wall elasticity, and sclerosis. They contribute to cardiovascular autonomic dysfunction with loss of vessel wall elasticity, peripheral vascular insufficiency, and impairment of nerve function [4].

AGEs reduce the flexibility and solubility of collagen, accelerating the fibrotic process, leading to aging and suppression of the immune system [5]. AGEs are also responsible for decreased keratinocyte proliferation, differentiation, and migration [6]. These factors often lead to poor wound healing and recurrent infections.

5.3 Cutaneous Manifestations Associated with Complications of Diabetes (Vascular and Neurological Damage)

5.3.1 Diabetic Dermopathy

Diabetic Dermopathy (DD), or pigmented pretibial patches or diabetic shin spots, is the most common dermatologic manifestation of diabetes. It has a strong predilection for pretibial skin in men older than 50 years of age [7] and may present in almost 50% diabetics [1]. It is often a late complication of long-standing diabetes and is associated with nephropathy, neuropathy, and retinopathy [8]. The pathogenesis is unclear; however, trauma, hemosiderin and melanin deposition, microangiopathic changes, and destruction of subcutaneous nerves have all been implicated [9, 10].

It is characterized by the presence of bilaterally symmetrical, asymptomatic, round, dull-red papules on bony prominences that progressively evolve into well-circumscribed, atrophic, brown macules with fine scaling over a few weeks. These eventually resolve with atrophy and hyperpigmentation over the next period of 1.5–2 years. At a particular time, different lesions can be seen in various stages of evolution. The pretibial area is the most commonly involved site, followed by forearms, lateral malleoli, or thighs. Histology of DD is nonspecific and epidermal edema, perivascular lymphocytic infiltrate, dilated papillary dermal vessels, and hemosiderin deposits can be observed depending on the stage of the lesion. Treatment is often not required as it is asymptomatic and self-resolving (Table 5.4).

5.3.2 Rubeosis Faciei

It is characterized by chronic erythema of the face or neck with a few telangiectasias in patients with Fitzpatrick skin type I to IV. The underlying pathogenesis is microangiopathic changes and small vessel dilation. The prevalence ranges from 7% in the community to 50% in hospitalized patients. It is often a sign of suboptimal

Table 5.4 Characteristics of specific cutaneous disorders associated with diabetes mellitus

Condition	Prevalence	Appearance	Characteristic distribution	Treatment
Diabetic dermopathy	Common	Small, brown, round to ovoid atrophic papules	Bilateral, asymmetric, pretibial	Not required
bullous diabeticorum	Rare <2%	Tense bullae on normal-appearing skin	Unilateral, acral distal surfaces of lower extremities	Conservative, drainage and prevention of secondary infection
Scleredema diabeticorum	2–10%	Thickening and induration of skin, peau d'orange appearance	Neck and upper back, symmetric	Generally unsatisfactory, PUVA and electron-beam therapy are most effective
Necrobiosis lipoidica	Rare	Ovoid hyperpigmented plaques with yellow-brown atrophic center and telangiectasis	Pretibial, bilateral or unilateral	Generally unsatisfactory, T optical and intralesional steroids are first-line
Generalised granuloma annulare	Rare	Multiple, asymptomatic, papules which coalesce to form annular rings with elevated border	Trunk and extremities	Steroids, PUVA, Dapsone all have been tried

glycaemic control [11] and retinopathy, neuropathy, and nephropathy can be associated with it [2]. There is no specific treatment; however, it may improve with better glycemic control and reduction of alcohol and caffeine intake.

5.3.3 *Palmar Erythema*

It presents with asymptomatic symmetric redness and warmth involving the hypothenar and thenar eminences of the palms. Microvascular changes in diabetes can lead to palmar erythema [12].

5.3.4 *Periungual Telangiectasias*

They arise due to venous capillary dilatation that occurs secondary to diabetic microangiopathy and may be seen in up to 50% of diabetics [13] and represent an early manifestation of diabetes-related microangiopathy [14]. It presents as asymptomatic erythema and telangiectasias surrounding the proximal nail folds.

5.3.5 Diabetic Foot Syndrome

Diabetic Foot Syndrome (DFS) is a significant cause of morbidity, mortality, and hospitalization in patients with diabetes. The incidence and prevalence of DFS ranges from 1–4% to 15–25%, respectively in patients with diabetes [15]. Neuropathy [16], atherosclerosis, peripheral ishaemia [16], and impaired wound healing play an important role in the development of DFS [17].

The clinical manifestations of DFS can range from callosities to chronic ulcers and foot malformations. The ulcers are mostly observed on trauma-prone sites and bony prominences such as toes, forefoot, and ankles. Diabetic neuro-osteoarthropathy or Charcot's foot is an irreversible deforming disease with progressive destruction of weight-bearing bones and joints. Charcot's foot presents with swelling of the ankle joint, the collapse of the midfoot arch, and clawing of the toes. Well-defined erysipelas-like erythema of the legs and feet can occur as a result of microangiopathy and may herald the onset of Charcot arthropathy.

Diabetes patients can also suffer from erythromelalgia with redness, warmth, and burning pain in the feet. The symptoms worsen with heat exposure and improve with cooling [18]. Wet gangrene can arise from sudden loss of perfusion to the already compromised cutaneous microcirculation and is a late manifestation of diabetic microangiopathy.

The prevention of foot ulcers includes daily surveillance, appropriate foot hygiene, proper footwear, walkers, or other devices to minimize and distribute pressure, parring of calluses, and liberal use of emollients. Hydrogels, hyperbaric oxygen therapy, topical growth factors, biofabricated skin grafts, topical and oral antibiotics have all been tried for improvement in diabetic foot ulcers [15]. Treatment of underlying ischemia plays an important role in patients with treatment-resistant or recurrent ulcers (Fig. 5.1).

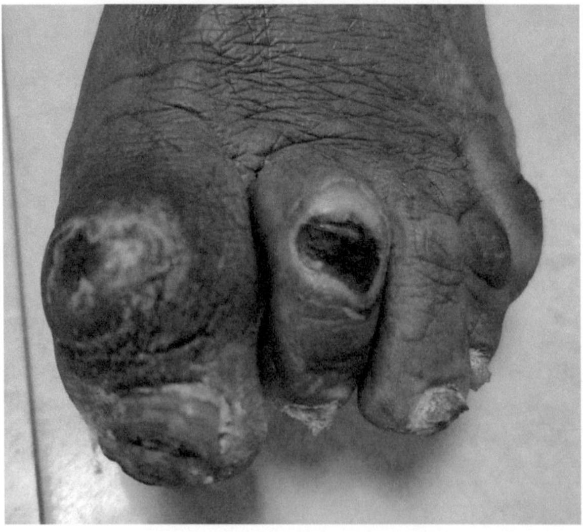

Fig. 5.1 Ulceration at the heads of metatarsals of first and second toes and toenail onychomycosis in a diabetic patient

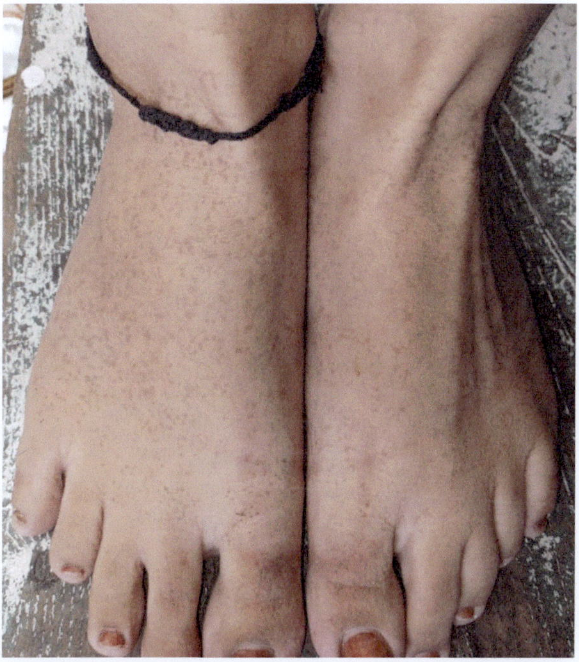

Fig. 5.2 Pigmented purpuric dermatosis

5.3.6 Pigmented Purpuric Dermatoses

It is seen in elderly diabetics and often coexists with diabetic dermopathy [19]. They are due to microvascular damage to capillaries and subsequent erythrocyte deposition [2]. They present as asymptomatic, non-blanching hyperpigmented macules and patches on pretibial areas and dorsum of the feet (Fig. 5.2).

5.4 Cutaneous Infections in Diabetes Mellitus

The prevalence of cutaneous infections is estimated to be 20–35% in patients with diabetes [5]. Micro-angiopathy, neuropathy, oxidative stress, abnormalities in leukocyte adherence, chemotaxis, and phagocytosis, and glucose-rich environment facilitates the growth of pathogens leading to chronic and recurrent skin infections.

5.4.1 Bacterial Infections

Staphylococcal and streptococcal infections such are recurrent folliculitis, furunculosis, carbuncles, erysipelas, and cellulitis are common in diabetic patients [20]. Methicillin-resistant Staphylococcus aureus (MRSA) colonization is also more common in diabetics as compared to non-diabetics and should be considered while treating the above cutaneous infections [21]. Other cutaneous infections such as green nail syndrome and erythrasma have also been frequently reported in diabetics [22]. Life-threatening infections such as necrotizing fasciitis, Fournier's gangrene, malignant otitis externa although rare, are more prevalent in diabetics [23].

5.4.2 Fungal Infections

Candidal infection Candidal infection can involve the mucosa (e.g. thrush, vulvovaginitis), intertriginous areas (e.g. intertrigo, erosio-interdigital, balanitis), or nails (e.g. onychomycosis, paronychia). Elevated salivary glucose concentrations [24] and elevated skin surface pH in skin folds [25] promote the growth of candida (Fig. 5.3).

Dermatophyte infections Dermatophyte infections are more prevalent among patients with diabetes [26]. Benign dermatophyte infections like tinea pedis can lead to serious consequences such as secondary bacterial infection, fungemia, or sepsis in diabetics and should be treated appropriately [27].

Systemic fungal infections such as rhino-orbital-cerebral mucormycosis, histoplasmosis aspergillosis, etc. are more common in patients with uncontrolled diabetes mellitus (Fig. 5.4).

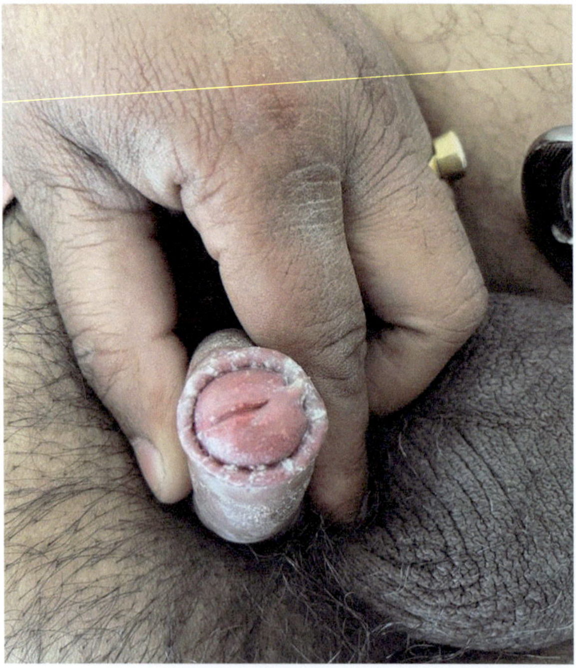

Fig. 5.3 Candidal balanoposthitis

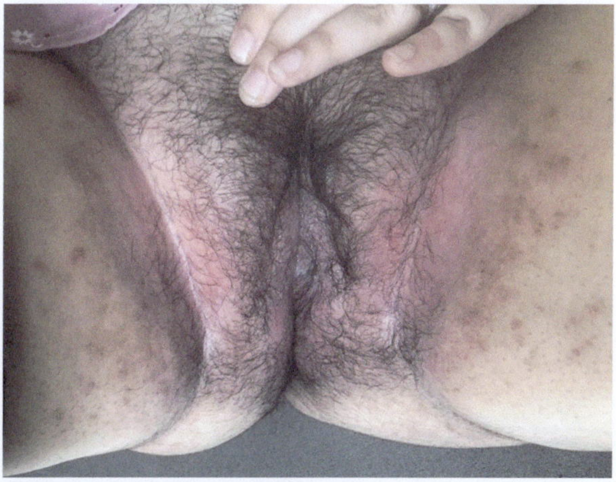

Fig. 5.4 Vulvovaginal candidiasis

5.5 Skin Diseases Associated with Insulin Resistance, Obesity and Metabolic Syndrome (Table 5.5)

5.5.1 *Acanthosis Nigricans*

Acanthosis nigricans (AN) is more common in patients with metabolic syndrome and type 2 diabetes mellitus [28]. Hyperinsulinemia activates insulin growth factor receptors-1 (IGF-1) on keratinocytes and fibroblasts and induces their proliferation, resulting in AN [29]. It presents as asymptomatic, bilaterally symmetrical, dark-brown velvety hyperpigmented plaques on intertriginous or flexural surfaces such as the back of the neck, axilla, elbows, inframammary creases, umbilicus, hands or groin. Histopathology shows hyperkeratosis, epidermal acanthosis, and papillomatosis without an increase in melanin or melanocytes. Treatment includes dietary modifications, increased physical activity, and weight reduction. Topical keratolytics such as ammonium lactate, salicylic acid, retinoids or oral retinoids, and metformin have been used in the treatment of AN [30, 31] (Fig. 5.5).

5.5.2 *Eruptive Xanthomas (EX)*

Lipid abnormalities are present in up to 75% of patients with diabetes [32]. EX can be seen in 2% of the patients with DM and are more common with type 2 DM. EX can appear in patients with DM with moderately raised triglyceride levels also. Hyperinsulinemia decreased lipoprotein lipase activity resulting in the accumulation of chylomicrons and other triglyceride-rich lipoproteins [33]. They present as asymptomatic, small grouped yellow-pink papules on extensor surfaces of the extremities, the buttocks. Koebnerisation can be present. Histopathology shows

Table 5.5 Skin manifestations of insulin resistance

Condition	Prevalence	Clinical manifestations	Distribution	Treatment
Acrochordons	Common	Soft, pedunculated skin-colored to hyperpigmented papules	Intertriginous areas (neck, axillae, and groin)	Excision, electrosurgery, cryotherapy
Acanthosis nigricans	Common	Symmetrical, velvety, light brown to black thickened plaques and accentuation of skin marks	Knuckles, intertriginous areas (neck, axillae, elbows, groin)	Lifestyle changes, oral or topical retinoids, ammonium lactate lactic acid
Eruptive xanthoma	Rare	Asymptomatic, small grouped yellow-pink papules	Extensor surfaces of the extremities, buttocks	Reduction in serum triglyceride levels and improving glycemic control

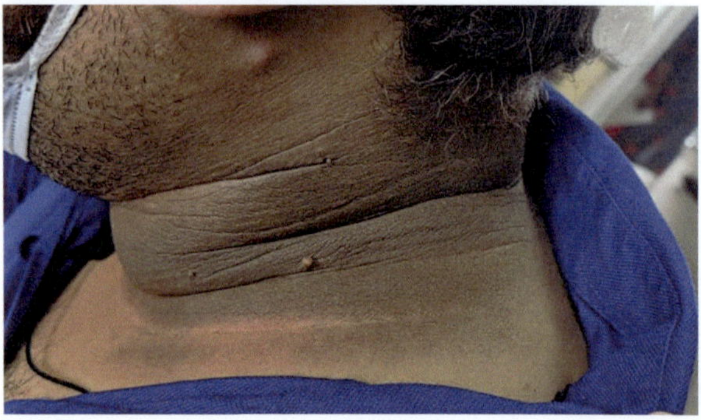

Fig. 5.5 Acanthosis nigricans and acrochordons

mixed inflammatory infiltrate and foam cells (lipid-laden macrophages) in the dermis. Treatment includes a reduction in serum triglyceride levels using fibrates, omega-3-fatty acids and improving glycemic control [34].

5.5.3 Acrochordons

Acrochordons (also known as soft benign fibromas, fibroepithelial polyps, or skin tags) are benign, soft, pedunculated growths that vary in size and can occur singularly or in groups. The neck, axilla, and periorbital area are most frequently involved, although other intertriginous areas can also be affected. Skin tags are common in the general population but are more prevalent in those with increased weight or age, and women. It has been reported that as many as three out of four patients presenting with acrochordons also have diabetes mellitus [35]. Excision, electrocautery, cryotherapy or ablative laser can be used for treatment.

5.6 Skin Manifestations Associated with Diabetes

5.6.1 Granulomatous Disorders

(a) **Necrobiosis Lipoidica**

Necrobiosis lipoidica (NL) is a chronic, disfiguring granulomatous disease seen in less than 1% of diabetics [36]. It is more common in diabetic as compared to non-diabetics [36]. The disease generally presents a decade or two later in type 2 diabetics as compared to type 1 [36] and pretibial skin in women is the commonest site of involvement [37]. The pathogenesis is complex wherein microangiopathy collagen dysregulation, abnormalities in neutrophil chemotaxis have been hypothesized to play a role [2, 36].

NL present as multiple erythematous papules that coalesce to form plaques with yellow-brown atrophic center with telangiectasias and red-brown borders on the pretibial areas. Other areas such as forearm, abdomen, scalp, and face can also be involved. The lesions are often asymptomatic; however, pruritus, hypoesthesia can be present. Ulceration can develop in one-third of lesions and has been associated with pain, secondary infections, and development of squamous cell carcinoma. The lesions can be bilateral and koebnerisation may be present. Histology shows palisading granulomatous inflammation with necrobiosis of collagen, mixed inflammatory infiltrate, decreased mucin and vessel wall thickening.

Various modalities have been used for the treatment of NL with varying degrees of success. Corticosteroids (oral, topical, or intralesional) are the most frequently used in the active stage of the disease. Other therapies include calcineurin inhibitors, pentoxifylline, antimalarials (e.g. hydroxychloroquine), PUVA, granulocyte colony-stimulating factor, dipyridamole, low-dose aspirin, and anti-tumor necrosis factor inhibitors (e.g. infliximab) [36]. Appropriate wound care is important for ulcerated lesions and includes topical antibiotics, protecting from further injury, and compression bandaging. Good glycaemic control is not beneficial in improving the skin lesions of NL.

(b) **Generalized Granuloma Annulare (GGA)**

Amongst various types of GA, only GGA is associated with diabetes. Less than 1% of patients with diabetes present with GGA; however, 10–15% of patients with GGA have diabetes [38]. It is more common in women in the fifth decade and those with type1 diabetes [38]. It presents with multiple, asymptomatic, skin-colored to erythematous, firm papules which coalesce and centrally involute to form hypo- or hyper-pigmented annular rings with elevated borders. The trunk and extremities are commonly involved. Histopathology shows dermal granulomatous inflammation surrounding foci of necrotic collagen and mucin. Corticosteroids, dapsone, cyclosporine, PUVA, antimalarials, retinoids, and calcineurin inhibitors all have been tried [39] (Fig. 5.6).

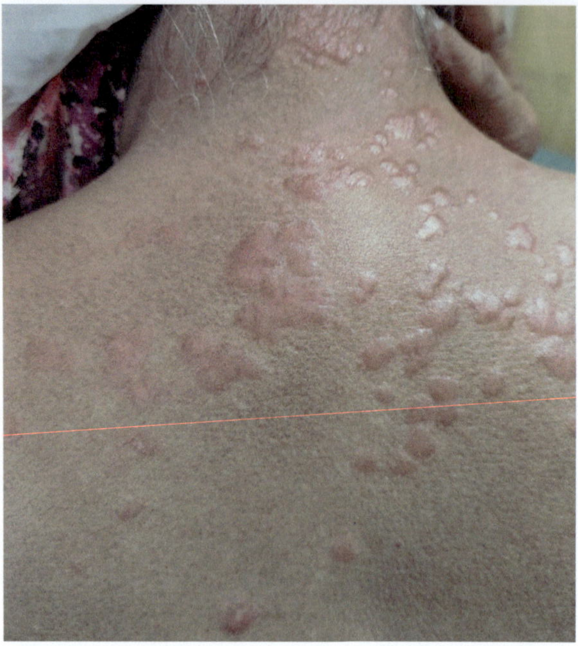

Fig. 5.6 Generalised granuloma annulare in a diabetic patient

5.6.2 Stiff Skin and Joints

(a) **Scleroderma-like Skin Changes**

Scleroderma-like skin change can be seen in 10–50% of patients with DM and is more common in those with type 1 DM and long-standing disease [40]. It is often associated with diabetic nephropathy and retinopathy and is believed to be caused by an increase in collagen in the upper dermis due to AGEs [41]. It presents as asymptomatic, bilaterally symmetrical, indurated, waxy-looking, thickened skin over acral areas specifically the dorsum of the fingers (sclerodactyly), proximal interphalangeal, and metacarpophalangeal joints. Less commonly, it can involve hands, arms, and back. It may be associated with diabetic hand syndrome which includes limited joint mobility, palmar fibromatosis (Dupuytren's contracture), and stenosing tenosynovitis ("trigger finger") [42]. Prayer sign which is the inability to press palmar surfaces on each hand together tightly may be positive. It can be differentiated from scleroderma by the absence of Raynaud's syndrome, pain, telangiectasia, and nail-fold capillary changes. In a few patients, the disease has a more early, aggressive course with truncal involvement. Histology shows increased thickness of the dermis, with minimal-to-absent mucin, and increased interlinking of collagen. Scleroderma-like skin changes are not associated with atrophy of the dermis, Raynaud's syndrome, pain, or telangiectasias which differentiates it from systemic sclerosis. Treatment is often unsatisfactory and includes improving glycemic control [43], aldose reductase inhibitors [43], and physiotherapy.

(b) **Limited Joint Mobility**

Diabetic cheiroarthropathy or limited Joint Mobility (LJM) is a common complication of long-standing DM. The majority of patients with LJM also present with scleroderma-like skin changes [44]. The prevalence of LJM is 4–26% in patients without diabetes and 8–58% in patients with diabetes [45]. The pathogenesis likely involves the hyperglycemia-induced formation of advanced glycation end-products, which accumulate to promote inflammation and the formation of stiffening cross-links between collagen [46]. It is commonly associated with other microvascular and macrovascular complications [46]. LJM presents with progressive flexed contractures and hindered joint extension, most commonly involving the metacarpophalangeal and interphalangeal joints of the hand. It often begins in the joints of the fifth finger thereafter gradually involving other joints of hands. Patients may present with an inability to press the palmar surfaces of each of their hands together (prayer sign) or against the surface of a table when their forearms are perpendicular to the surface of the table (tabletop sign) [47]. These changes occur as a result of periarticular enlargement of connective tissue. There are no curative treatments. Symptomatic patients may benefit from non-steroidal anti-inflammatory drugs or targeted injection of corticosteroids. LJM is best managed with improved glycemic control [48], as well as, regular stretching to maintain and minimize further limitations in joint mobility.

(c) **Scleredema Diabetocorum**

It is a chronic and slowly progressive sclerotic skin disorder seen in 2.5–14% of all patients with DM [49]. It is more common in women and patients with long-standing diseases [50]. Pathogenesis is poorly understood; however non-enzymatic glycosylation of collagen, increased production of collagen by fibroblasts, and decreased collagen breakdown are hypothesized to play a role [51].

It characteristically presents as asymptomatic, bilaterally symmetrical, slowly progressive thickening of the skin on the upper back, shoulders, and back of the neck. Other areas such as the face, chest, abdomen, buttocks, and thighs can also be involved; however, extremities are mostly spared. Patients with longstanding disease can develop a reduced range of motion in joints and restrictive respiratory problems. Histopathology shows increased collagen in the reticular dermis with a surrounding mucinous infiltrate, without any edema or sclerosis.

Various modalities such as corticosteroids, immunosuppressives, UVA1, PUVA, intravenous immunoglobulin, and electron-beam therapy have been tried but the results are often disappointing [52]. The improved blood sugar level is preventive but not therapeutic. Physiotherapy is the mainstay in those with long-standing diseases and helps in improving their quality of life.

(d) **Huntley's Papules**

They are mostly observed in patients with type 2 diabetes and maybe an early sign of diabetic thick skin [53]. They commonly present as asymptomatic, grouped, skin-colored papules coalescing to form plaques on the dorsal surface of the hands particularly over the metacarpophalangeal joints and periungual areas. Treatment is often not satisfactory and includes topical emollients, ammonium lactate, and retinoids [53].

5.6.3 Bullosis Diabeticorum

Bullosis diabeticorum (BD) is a rare blistering disease seen in 0.5–1% of diabetics with long-standing disease. It is mostly seen in males between 50 and 70 years of age and is commoner in those with type 1 diabetes who have vascular complications such as neuropathy, nephropathy, and retinopathy [54]. Pathogenesis is elusive and many theories such as autoimmune, UV exposure, AGEs, and changes in microvasculature have been proposed [55].

It presents with sudden-onset, non-tender, non-erythematous, firm, sterile bullae varying in size from 0.5 to 5 cm present on acral areas of the lower extremities without any history of trauma to the affected area Histopathology shows an intraepidermal or subepidermal bulla with spongiosis and minimal inflammatory infiltrate, and normal immunofluorescence. They resolve on their own in 2–6 weeks in the absence of any secondary infections.

5.6.4 Acquired Perforating Dermatosis

Acquired perforating dermatoses (APD) are commonly associated with chronic renal failure and diabetes [56]. The prevalence of APD in diabetes mellitus is estimated to be around 15% [57]. Various hypotheses have been implicated in the development of APD which includes repetitive superficial trauma, epidermal or dermal metabolic derangements, microvascular abnormalities, and accumulation of immunogenic substances [56].

It presents as pruritic, bilaterally symmetrical, hyperkeratotic umbilicated-papules and nodules with centralized keratin plugs on extensors surface of arms and legs. Koebnerization is often seen and the lesions with hyperpigmentation. Histology shows the absence or degeneration of dermal connective tissue components (e.g. collagen, elastic fibers), transepidermal extrusion of keratotic material, and lymphocytic infiltrate.

The management includes topical keratolytics, retinoids, high-potency corticosteroids, and pruritus relief [58]. Generalized lesions may require oral retinoids, PUVA, oral antibiotics such as doxycycline, allopurinol, or cryotherapy [58]. Improvement in glycemic control plays an essential role in management (Fig. 5.7).

5.6.5 Other Miscellaneous Disorders

(a) **Ichthyosis**

Acquired ichthyosis has been reported in 22–48% of patients with type 1 DM [59]. AGEs and microangiopathy are believed to play a role. It presents

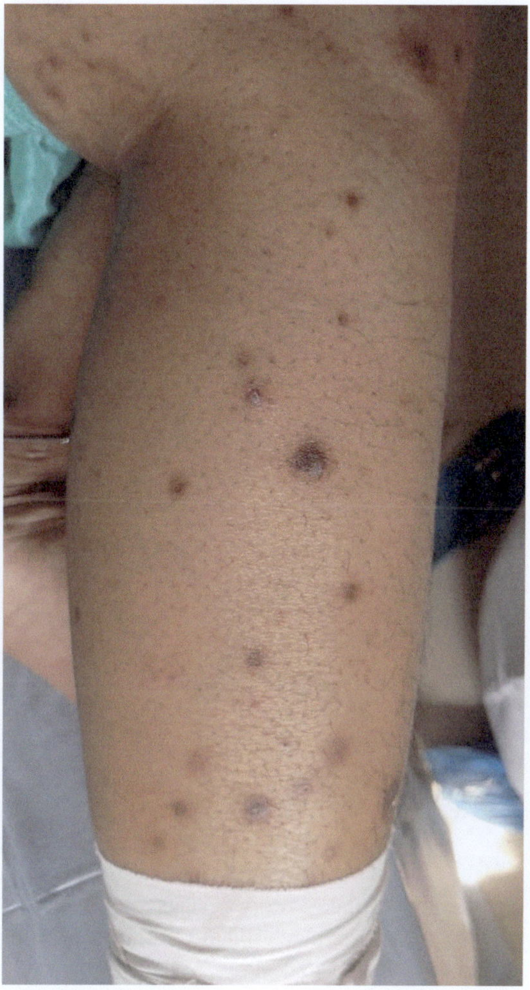

Fig. 5.7 Acquired perforating dermatosis on the legs

with dryness and scaling on the anterior shin and less commonly hands or feet. Treatment includes topical emollients or keratolytic agents [60] (Fig. 5.8).

(b) **Xerosis**

Xerosis or dry skin is one of the commonest cutaneous manifestations, seen in almost half of the patients with diabetes [61]. It is seen in the feet of patients with diabetes. Treatment includes topical emollients and avoidance of cracks, fissures, and secondary infections [62].

(c) **Pruritus**

Diabetes patients can develop pruritus on the scalp, ankles, feet, trunk, or genitalia [63]. It is more frequent in those with xerosis and neuropathy.

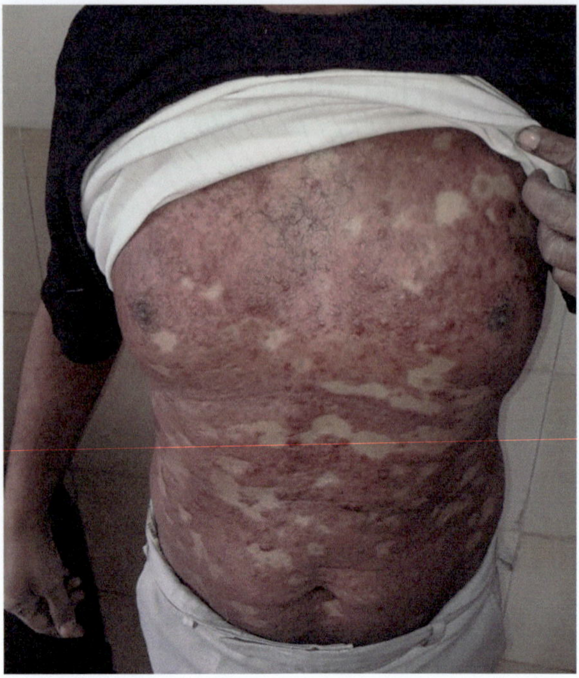

Fig. 5.8 Multiple tense vesicles and bulla on an urticated base on trunk and extremities in a diabetic patients due to vildagliptin

Treatments include oral antihistaminic, topical capsaicin, topical lidocaine, and oral anticonvulsants (e.g. gabapentin or pregabalin).

(d) **Keratosis Pilaris**

The lesions occur more frequently and are disseminated in those with diabetes [40]. It presents as asymptomatic, keratotic perifollicular papules with erythema on the posterior surfaces of the upper arm, thighs, and buttocks. Treatments include topical keratolytics, emollients, and retinoids.

(e) **Yellow Skin and Nails**

It is observed in elderly patients with type 2 diabetes and arises due to the accumulation of various substances such as carotene or glycosylated proteins [11]. Clinical manifestations include asymptomatic yellow discolorations involving the palms, soles, face, or nails.

(f) **Psoriasis**

Psoriasis is associated with diabetes, hypertension, and metabolic syndrome [64]. Younger patients and those with severe psoriasis are also at risk of developing diabetes.

(g) **Lichen Planus**

Various studies have found an association between lichen planus and glucose abnormalities [65]. Also, patients with diabetes are more likely to develop oral lichen planus [65].

(h) **Vitiligo**

Vitiligo occurs more frequently in women and is also more common in type 1 than in type 2 diabetes mellitus [66]. Coinciding vitiligo and type 1 diabetes mellitus may be associated with endocrine autoimmune abnormalities of the gastric parietal cells, adrenal, or thyroid [67].

(i) **Hidradenitis Supparativa (HS)**

Diabetes is three times more common in patients with HS as compared to the normal population [68]. Therefore, HS patients should be screened for diabetes [69].

(j) **Glucagonoma**

Patients with glucagonoma can also have diabetes mellitus. In patients with glucagonoma, diabetes mellitus frequently presents before the development of necrolytic migratory erythema [70]. Approximately 20–40% of patients will present with diabetes mellitus before the diagnosis of glucagonoma [70]. Of those patients diagnosed with glucagonoma but not diabetes mellitus, 76–94% will eventually develop diabetes mellitus [71].

5.7 Cutaneous Changes Associated with Diabetes Medications (Table 5.6)

Table 5.6 Characteristics of cutaneous disorders associated with treatment of diabetes mellitus

Condition	Prevalence	Appearance	Characteristic distribution	Treatment
Lipohypertrophy	Common	Soft, rubbery, lipoma-like dermal nodules	Insulin injection sites	Rotation of injection sites Avoid injection to areas of lipohypertrophy
Lipoatrophy	Rare	Cutaneous depressions	Insulin injection sites	Rotation of injection sites, less common with synthetic insulin
Drug-induced bullous pemphigoid	Rare	Tense blisters on normal, erythematous, or urticarial skin	Generalized	Discontinuation of offending medication, oral steroid and dapsone

5.7.1 Insulin

Lipohypertrophy is characterized by localized adipocyte hypertrophy and presents with soft dermal nodules at insulin injection sites. It can lead to delayed insulin absorption and affects less than 30% of patients who use insulin [72]. It resolves over a few months on avoidance of the use of insulin at affected sites.

Lipoatrophy presents as round concave areas of adipose tissue atrophy on insulin injection sites. It is rare now with the introduction of modern purified forms of insulin.

Allergic reactions can arise due to hypersensitivity reactions to insulin itself or the additives. Systemic allergic reactions to insulin are rarely occurring in only 0.01% of patients [72]. Other skin changes associated with insulin use include erythema, pruritus, urticaria, induration, painful nodules, granulomas, nodular amyloidosis, calcification.

5.7.2 Oral Medications

DPP-IV inhibitors, such as vildagliptin, have been associated with bullous pemphigoid [73], Stevens-Johnson syndrome, and angioedema [74]. Allergic skin and photosensitivity reactions can occur with sulfonylureas [75]. Sulfonylureas, chlorpropamide, and tolbutamide are associated with the development of maculopapular rash in the initial few months of starting treatment which improves with the stoppage of the medication [75, 76]. Chlorpropamide can cause acute facial flushing following alcohol consumption in susceptible individuals [77]. Canagliflozin, an SGLT-2 inhibitor, has been associated with an increased risk of genital fungal infections [78].

References

1. Bustan RS, Wasim D, Yderstræde KB, Bygum A. Specific skin signs as a cutaneous marker of diabetes mellitus and the prediabetic state—a systematic review. Dan Med J. 2017;64(1):A5316.
2. Demirseren DD, Emre S, Akoglu G, Arpacı D, Arman A, Metin A, et al. Relationship between skin diseases and extracutaneous complications of diabetes mellitus: clinical analysis of 750 patients. Am J Clin Dermatol. 2014;15:65–70.
3. Camera A, Hopps E, Caimi G. Diabetic microangiopathy: physiopathological, clinical and therapeutic aspects. Minerva Endocrinol. 2007;32:209–29.
4. Ando A, Miyamoto M, Kotani K, Okada K, Nagasaka S, Ishibashi S. Cardio-ankle vascular index and indices of diabetic polyneuropathy in patients with type 2 diabetes. J Diabetes Res. 2017;2017:2810914.
5. de Macedo GM, Nunes S, Barreto T. Skin disorders in diabetes mellitus: an epidemiology and physiopathology review. Diabetol Metab Syndr. 2016;8:63.

6. Behm B, Schreml S, Landthaler M, Babilas P. Skin signs in diabetes mellitus. J Eur Acad Dermatol Venereol. 2012;26:1203–11.
7. Morgan AJ, Schwartz RA. Diabetic dermopathy: a subtle sign with grave implications. J Am Acad Dermatol. 2008;58:447–51.
8. Romano G, Moretti G, Di Benedetto A, Giofrè C, Di Cesare E, Russo G, et al. Skin lesions in diabetes mellitus: prevalence and clinical correlations. Diabetes Res Clin Pract. 1998;39:101–6.
9. Houck GM, Morgan MB. A reappraisal of the histologic findings of pigmented pretibial patches of diabetes mellitus. J Cutan Pathol. 2004;31:141–4.
10. McCash S, Emanuel PO. Defining diabetic dermopathy. J Dermatol. 2011;38:988–92.
11. Duff M, Demidova O, Blackburn S, Shubrook J. Cutaneous manifestations of diabetes mellitus. Clin Diabetes. 2015;33:40–8.
12. Serrao R, Zirwas M, English JC. Palmar erythema. Am J Clin Dermatol. 2007;8:347–56.
13. Landau J, Davis E. The small blood-vessels of the conjunctiva and nailbed in diabetes mellitus. Lancet. 1960;2:731–4.
14. Oumeish OY. Skin disorders in patients with diabetes. Clin Dermatol. 2008;26:235–42.
15. Amin N, Doupis J. Diabetic foot disease: from the evaluation of the "foot at risk" to the novel diabetic ulcer treatment modalities. World J Diabetes. 2016;7:153–64.
16. Jeffcoate WJ, Harding KG. Diabetic foot ulcers. Lancet. 2003;361:1545–51.
17. Lobmann R, Schultz G, Lehnert H. Proteases and the diabetic foot syndrome: mechanisms and therapeutic implications. Diabetes Care. 2005;28:461–71.
18. Davis MD, O'Fallon WM, Rogers RS III, Rooke TW. Natural history of erythromelalgia: presentation and outcome in 168 patients. Arch Dermatol. 2000;136:330–6.
19. Lithner F. Purpura, pigmentation and yellow nails of the lower extremities in diabetics. Acta Med Scand. 1976;199:203–8.
20. Casqueiro J, Casqueiro J, Alves C. Infections in patients with diabetes mellitus: a review of pathogenesis. Indian J Endocrinol Metab. 2012;16(Suppl 1):S27–36.
21. Kutlu SS, Cevahir N, Akalin S, Akin F, Dirgen Caylak S, Bastemir M, et al. Prevalence and risk factors for methicillin-resistant Staphylococcus aureus colonization in a diabetic outpatient population: a prospective cohort study. Am J Infect Control. 2012;40:365–8.
22. Driscoll JA, Brody SL, Kollef MH. The epidemiology, pathogenesis and treatment of Pseudomonas aeruginosa infections. Drugs. 2007;67:351–68.
23. Treviño González JL, Reyes Suárez LL, Hernández de León JE. Malignant otitis externa: an updated review. Am J Otolaryngol. 2021;42:102894.
24. Sashikumar R, Kannan R. Salivary glucose levels and oral candidal carriage in type II diabetics. Oral Surg Oral Med Oral Pathol Oral Radiol Endod. 2010;109:706–11.
25. Yosipovitch G, Tur E, Cohen O, Rusecki Y. Skin surface pH in intertriginous areas in NIDDM patients. Possible correlation to candidal intertrigo. Diabetes Care. 1993;16:560–3.
26. Saunte DM, Holgersen JB, Haedersdal M, Strauss G, Bitsch M, Svendsen OL, et al. Prevalence of toe nail onychomycosis in diabetic patients. Acta Derm Venereol. 2006;86:425–8.
27. Rich P. Onychomycosis and tinea pedis in patients with diabetes. J Am Acad Dermatol. 2000;43:S130–4.
28. Stuart CA, Gilkison CR, Smith MM, Bosma AM, Keenan BS, Nagamani M. Acanthosis nigricans as a risk factor for non-insulin dependent diabetes mellitus. Clin Pediatr (Phila). 1998;37:73–9.
29. Das A, Datta D, Kassir M, Wollina U, Galadari H, Lotti T, et al. Acanthosis nigricans: a review. J Cosmet Dermatol. 2020;19:1857–65.
30. Blobstein SH. Topical therapy with tretinoin and ammonium lactate for acanthosis nigricans associated with obesity. Cutis. 2003;71:33–4.
31. Higgins SP, Freemark M, Prose NS. Acanthosis nigricans: a practical approach to evaluation and management. Dermatol Online J. 2008;14:2.
32. Vergès B. Pathophysiology of diabetic dyslipidaemia: where are we? Diabetologia. 2015;58:886–99.

33. Merola JF, Mengden SJ, Soldano A, Rosenman K. Eruptive xanthomas. Dermatol Online J. 2008;14:10.
34. Zak A, Zeman M, Slaby A, Vecka M. Xanthomas: clinical and pathophysiological relations. Biomed Pap Med Fac Univ Palacky Olomouc Czech Repub. 2014;158:181–8.
35. Kahana M, Grossman E, Feinstein A, Ronnen M, Cohen M, Millet MS. Skin tags: a cutaneous marker for diabetes mellitus. Acta Derm Venereol. 1987;67:175–7.
36. Reid SD, Ladizinski B, Lee K, Baibergenova A, Alavi A. Update on necrobiosis lipoidica: a review of etiology, diagnosis, and treatment options. J Am Acad Dermatol. 2013;69:783–91.
37. O'Toole EA, Kennedy U, Nolan JJ, Young MM, Rogers S, Barnes L. Necrobiosis lipoidica: only a minority of patients have diabetes mellitus. Br J Dermatol. 1999;140:283–6.
38. Yun JH, Lee JY, Kim MK, Seo YJ, Kim MH, Cho KH, et al. Clinical and pathological features of generalized granuloma annulare with their correlation: a retrospective multicenter study in Korea. Ann Dermatol. 2009;21:113–9.
39. Cyr PR. Diagnosis and management of granuloma annulare. Am Fam Physician. 2006;74:1729–34.
40. Yosipovitch G, Hodak E, Vardi P, Shraga I, Karp M, Sprecher E, et al. The prevalence of cutaneous manifestations in IDDM patients and their association with diabetes risk factors and microvascular complications. Diabetes Care. 1998;21:506–9.
41. Haustein UF. Scleroderma-like lesions in insulin-dependent diabetes mellitus. J Eur Acad Dermatol Venereol. 1999;13:50–3.
42. Yosipovitch G, Yosipovitch Z, Karp M, Mukamel M. Trigger finger in young patients with insulin dependent diabetes. J Rheumatol. 1990;17:951–2.
43. Yosipovitch G, Loh KC, Hock OB. Medical pearl: scleroderma-like skin changes in patients with diabetes mellitus. J Am Acad Dermatol. 2003;49:109–11.
44. Sawatkar GU, Kanwar AJ, Dogra S, Bhadada SK, Dayal D. Spectrum of cutaneous manifestations of type 1 diabetes mellitus in 500 South Asian patients. Br J Dermatol. 2014;171:1402–6.
45. Gerrits EG, Landman GW, Nijenhuis-Rosien L, Bilo HJ. Limited joint mobility syndrome in diabetes mellitus: a minireview. World J Diabetes. 2015;6:1108–12.
46. Labad J, Rozadilla A, Garcia-Sancho P, Nolla JM, Montanya E. Limited joint mobility progression in type 1 diabetes: a 15-year follow-up study. Int J Endocrinol. 2018;2018:1897058.
47. Fitzgibbons PG, Weiss AP. Hand manifestations of diabetes mellitus. J Hand Surg Am. 2008;33:771–5.
48. Lindsay JR, Kennedy L, Atkinson AB, Bell PM, Carson DJ, McCance DR, et al. Reduced prevalence of limited joint mobility in type 1 diabetes in a U.K. clinic population over a 20-year period. Diabetes Care. 2005;28:658–61.
49. Rongioletti F, Kaiser F, Cinotti E, Metze D, Battistella M, Calzavara-Pinton PG, et al. Scleredema. A multicentre study of characteristics, comorbidities, course and therapy in 44 patients. J Eur Acad Dermatol Venereol. 2015;29:2399–404.
50. Cole GW, Headley J, Skowsky R. Scleredema diabeticorum: a common and distinct cutaneous manifestation of diabetes mellitus. Diabetes Care. 1983;6:189–92.
51. Martín C, Requena L, Manrique K, Manzarbeitia FD, Rovira A. Scleredema diabeticorum in a patient with type 2 diabetes mellitus. Case Rep Endocrinol. 2011;2011:560273.
52. Ferreli C, Gasparini G, Parodi A, Cozzani E, Rongioletti F, Atzori L. Cutaneous manifestations of scleroderma and scleroderma-like disorders: a comprehensive review. Clin Rev Allergy Immunol. 2017;53:306–36.
53. Guarneri C, Guarneri F, Borgia F, Vaccaro M. Finger pebbles in a diabetic patient: Huntley's papules. Int J Dermatol. 2005;44:755–6.
54. Larsen K, Jensen T, Karlsmark T, Holstein PE. Incidence of bullosis diabeticorum—a controversial cause of chronic foot ulceration. Int Wound J. 2008;5:591–6.
55. Lipsky BA, Baker PD, Ahroni JH. Diabetic bullae: 12 cases of a purportedly rare cutaneous disorder. Int J Dermatol. 2000;39:196–200.
56. Saray Y, Seçkin D, Bilezikçi B. Acquired perforating dermatosis: clinicopathological features in twenty-two cases. J Eur Acad Dermatol Venereol. 2006;20:679–88.

57. Poliak SC, Lebwohl MG, Parris A, Prioleau PG. Reactive perforating collagenosis associated with diabetes mellitus. N Engl J Med. 1982;306:81–4.
58. Van Hattem S, Bootsma AH, Thio HB. Skin manifestations of diabetes. Cleve Clin J Med. 2008;75:772, 4, 6–7 passim.
59. Pavlović MD, Milenković T, Dinić M, Misović M, Daković D, Todorović S, et al. The prevalence of cutaneous manifestations in young patients with type 1 diabetes. Diabetes Care. 2007;30:1964–7.
60. Patel N, Spencer LA, English JC III, Zirwas MJ. Acquired ichthyosis. J Am Acad Dermatol. 2006;55:647–56.
61. Goyal A, Raina S, Kaushal SS, Mahajan V, Sharma NL. Pattern of cutaneous manifestations in diabetes mellitus. Indian J Dermatol. 2010;55:39–41.
62. Pavicic T, Korting HC. Xerosis and callus formation as a key to the diabetic foot syndrome: dermatologic view of the problem and its management. J Dtsch Dermatol Ges. 2006;4:935–41.
63. Yamaoka H, Sasaki H, Yamasaki H, Ogawa K, Ohta T, Furuta H, et al. Truncal pruritus of unknown origin may be a symptom of diabetic polyneuropathy. Diabetes Care. 2010;33:150–5.
64. Armstrong AW, Harskamp CT, Armstrong EJ. Psoriasis and the risk of diabetes mellitus: a systematic review and meta-analysis. JAMA Dermatol. 2013;149:84–91.
65. Seyhan M, Ozcan H, Sahin I, Bayram N, Karincaoğlu Y. High prevalence of glucose metabolism disturbance in patients with lichen planus. Diabetes Res Clin Pract. 2007;77:198–202.
66. Mendes AL, Miot HA, Haddad VJ. Diabetes mellitus and the skin. An Bras Dermatol. 2017;92:8–20.
67. Van den Driessche A, Eenkhoorn V, Van Gaal L, De Block C. Type 1 diabetes and autoimmune polyglandular syndrome: a clinical review. Neth J Med. 2009;67:376–87.
68. Phan K, Charlton O, Smith SD. Hidradenitis suppurativa and diabetes mellitus: updated systematic review and adjusted meta-analysis. Clin Exp Dermatol. 2019;44:e126–32.
69. Bui TL, Silva-Hirschberg C, Torres J, Armstrong AW. Hidradenitis suppurativa and diabetes mellitus: a systematic review and meta-analysis. J Am Acad Dermatol. 2018;78:395–402.
70. Wermers RA, Fatourechi V, Wynne AG, Kvols LK, Lloyd RV. The glucagonoma syndrome. Clinical and pathologic features in 21 patients. Medicine (Baltimore). 1996;75:53–63.
71. Halvorson SA, Gilbert E, Hopkins RS, Liu H, Lopez C, Chu M, et al. Putting the pieces together: necrolytic migratory erythema and the glucagonoma syndrome. J Gen Intern Med. 2013;28:1525–9.
72. Richardson T, Kerr D. Skin-related complications of insulin therapy: epidemiology and emerging management strategies. Am J Clin Dermatol. 2003;4:661–7.
73. Attaway A, Mersfelder TL, Vaishnav S, Baker JK. Bullous pemphigoid associated with dipeptidyl peptidase IV inhibitors. A case report and review of literature. J Dermatol Case Rep. 2014;8:24–8.
74. Byrd JS, Minor DS, Elsayed R, Marshall GD. DPP-4 inhibitors and angioedema: a cause for concern? Ann Allergy Asthma Immunol. 2011;106:436–8.
75. Hitselberger JF, Fosnaugh RP. Photosensitivity due to chlorpropamide. JAMA. 1962;180:62–3.
76. Walker G, Slater JD, Westlake EK, Nabarro JD. Clinical experience with tolbutamide. Br Med J. 1957;2:323–5.
77. Leslie RD, Pyke DA. Chlorpropamide-alcohol flushing: a dominantly inherited trait associated with diabetes. Br Med J. 1978;2:1519–21.
78. Nyirjesy P, Sobel JD, Fung A, Mayer C, Capuano G, Ways K, et al. Genital mycotic infections with canagliflozin, a sodium glucose co-transporter 2 inhibitor, in patients with type 2 diabetes mellitus: a pooled analysis of clinical studies. Curr Med Res Opin. 2014;30:1109–19.

Chapter 6
Pathophysiology of PCOS

Priyadarshini Sahu, Nidhi Sharma, and Amalia Tsiatoura

6.1 Introduction

Polycystic ovarian disease (PCOD) was originally described by Stein and Leventhal in females who presented with amenorrhoea/oligomenorrhoea, hirsutism, obesity, infertility and bilateral polycystic ovaries. Now-a-days, various metabolic diseases are associated with PCOD and is known as PCOS (polycystic ovarian syndrome). It is also known as Hyperandrogenic anovulation (HA) or Stein Leventhal syndrome. It is the most common endocrine disorder, that affect approximately 15% women in their child-bearing age group. It has been observed in women of reproductive age group among all the cultures and ethnicity. This chapter reviews the pathophysiology of PCOS.

6.2 Definition of PCOS

There are various criteria to diagnose PCOS, which includes 1990 National Institutes of Health (NIH) criteria, 2003 Rotterdam criteria, 2006 Androgen excess & PCOS (AE-PCOS) society criteria and 2007 Japan Society of Obstetrics and Gynaecology (JSOG) criteria (Japan) [1, 2]. Among all these, Rotterdam criteria is mostly used to

P. Sahu (✉)
Consultant Dermatologist, Department of Telemedicine, PGIMER, Chandigarh, India

N. Sharma
Skin Health clinic, Gurugram, Haryana, India

A. Tsiatoura
Cosmetic Derma Medicine Center, Athens, Greece

R. Singh, N. Sharma (eds.), *A Guide to Hormonal Dermatology*,
https://doi.org/10.1007/978-981-99-7715-4_6

diagnose patients of PCOS. The Rotterdam criteria [3] require at least two out of the following three characteristics to be present for a diagnosis of PCOS to be made: clinical and/or biochemical hyperandrogenism, ovulatory dysfunction, and polycystic ovarian morphology (PCOM). Clinical features of hyperandrogenism includes hirsutism, acne, seborrhoea, acanthosis nigricans and alopecia. On investigations high levels of luteinizing hormone, manifesting as oligomenorrhea or amenorrhea. Ultrasonography shows polycystic ovaries, charaterized by presence of $\geq$12 follicles in ovary and with follicle size ranging between 2 and 9 mm, ovarian volume $\geq$10 mL. Recently it has been associated with metabolic syndrome such as obesity, insulin resistance and type 2 diabetes mellitus.

6.3 Phenotypes

Patients of PCOS are divided into four phenotypes based on their presentation [4]:

(a) Frank or classic polycystic ovary PCOS (chronic anovulation/oligomenorrhea, hyperandrogenism, and polycystic ovaries)
(b) Classic non-polycystic ovary PCOS (chronic anovulation, hyperandrogenism, and normal ovaries)
(c) Ovulatory PCOS (regular menstrual cycles, hyperandrogenism, and polycystic ovaries)
(d) Mild or normo-androgenic PCOS (chronic anovulation, normal androgens, and polycystic ovaries)

The females with oligomenorrhea/chronic anovulation with hyperandrogenism have higher risks of insulin resistance, diabetes, cardiovascular disease, endometrial dysfunction, and pregnancy complications [3]. Whereas, females with Normo-androgenic and Ovulatory PCOS have lower risk of chronic diseases as judged by lower incidences of abdominal obesity, insulin resistance, and inflammation [5, 6]. Moreover, women with Ovulatory PCOS appear to have lower risks of endometrial carcinoma [7].

6.4 Pathophysiology of PCOS

Hyperandrogenism is the prime feature of PCOS, primarily from the excess production from the ovaries and adrenals. The key feature is hyperandrogenism, which has a synergistic effect with insulin resistance to induce the development of PCOS. There is a variation in individual contributions of hyperandrogenism and insulin resistance differ from patient to patient, which accounts for the heterogenous nature of PCOS and its presentation. There is a vicious cycle comprise of hyperandrogenism, ovulatory dysfunction, aberrant gonadotropin-releasing hormone (GnRH) pulsation and the resulting abnormal gonadotropin secretion, and insulin resistance. All these factors interact and exacerbate each other.

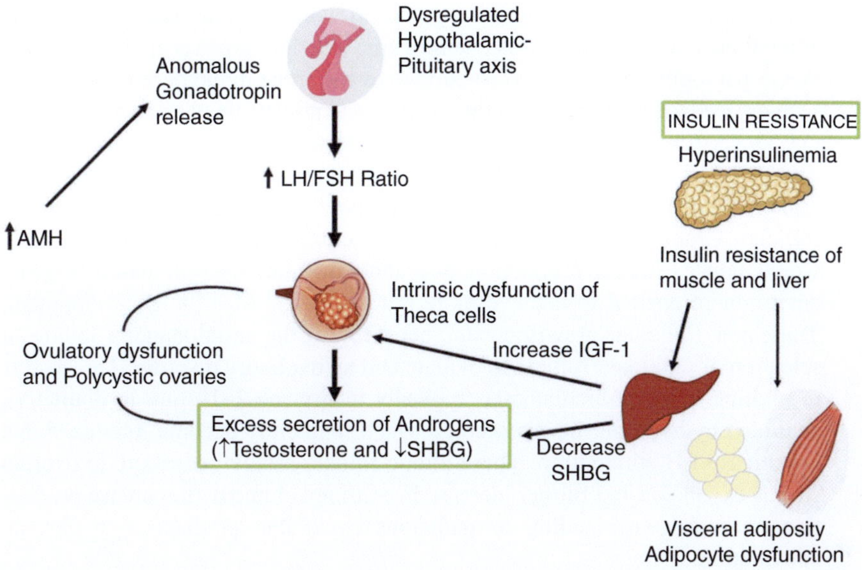

Fig. 6.1 Diagram representing PCOS Pathophysiology. The vicious cycle comprises of hyperandrogenism, abnormal secretion of gonadotrophin and insulin resistance. Key feature is excess androgen secretion, which has a synergistic effect on insulin resistance and aggravates hyperinsulinemia. Hyperinsulinemia act on theca cells and increases androgen secretion. It also inhibits SHBG in the liver, hence increasing the circulating concentration of free testosterone. In addition, Insulin resistance causes visceral adiposity and adipocyte dysfunction especially in liver and muscle. The anomalous secretion of gonadotropin is characterized by a high LH/ FSH ratio, which induces ovarian dysfunction, and again leads to hypersecretion of androgens. Further, the high concentration of AMH, further exacerbates the ovarian dysfunction

The origin of this vicious cycle of PCOS remains unknown. The simplest explanation for this complex and heterogeneous syndrome would be that hyperandrogenism is a predisposing factor, while insulin resistance triggers the development of PCOS (Fig. 6.1).

(a) Pituitary dysfunction: There is an increase in amplitude and frequency of GnRH pulsation that leads to increase in LH secretion. Elevation in LH secretion with increase in LH/FSH ratio is a hallmark of PCOS.
(b) Increase ovarian androgen production: The primary mechanism responsible for hyperandrogenism includes abnormal LH secretory dynamics and hyperinsulinemia due to insulin resistance, which further potentiate the action of LH. Abnormal increase in LH production affect the thecal cells of ovaries resulting in overproduction of androgens. However, in some patients there is normal level of LH levels, but still have increased levels of androgens. This may be due overexpression of genes such as CYP17, CYP11a, CYP21 and CYP19. These genes cause an intrinsic dysfunction of key ovarian steroidogenic enzyme especially 3b-hydroxysteroid dehydrogenase (3b-HSD) and 17,20-lyase. Hypersecretion of androgens is associated with aberrant follicular growth and ovarian dysfunction. Adrenal androgen production (i.e., androstenedione,

DHEA, DHEA-S) is also increased in PCOS women. Androgens produced by adrenal have no or little intrinsic androgenic activity, however it contributes to PCOS pathophysiology via conversion to testosterone in the periphery.

Increased local androgen production leads to polycystic ovarian morphology via conversion to potent 5α-reduced androgens. It can not be aromatized to estrogen and further cannot inhibit both FSH induction of LH receptors on granulosa cells and aromatase activity, thus leads to progressive development of follicles. Granulosa cells are sensitive to insulin like growth factors and FSH, which induce estrogen production, but cannot maintain the follicular estrogenic environment needed to achieve more advance stage of follicle development. Thus, new follicular growth occurs, but arrest at the antral stage; a failure of selection of dominant follicle to ovulate and an ovulatory disorder. This results in multiple small follicular cyst (typically measuring 2–10 mm in diameter), encircled by hyperplastic theca cells, which frequently become luteinized due to increase LH stimulation. These atretic follicle finally contribute to ovarian stroma expansion and further increase in ovarian volume with increase production of androgens, leading to malicious cycle that predispose to chronic anovulation.

(c) Role of Insulin: Insulin insensitivity is a common feature in obese as compared to lean women with PCOS. Its overall prevalence ranges from 50% to 75%. Increased circulating insulin levels cause hyperandrogenism by two main mechanisms, firstly by stimulating ovarian androgens productions and secondly by inhibiting SHBG and IGFBP-1 production in the liver. Insulin also increases the amplitude, not the frequency of LH pulses at pituitary level. By decreasing SHBG and IGFBP-1, it increases circulating level of androgens and IGF-1 (Insulin like growth factor 1). Of the total androgens produced only 1% circulates freely. Rest 99% are in the bound form, 80% bound to sex hormone binding globulin (SHBG) and 18% to the albumin. In PCOS patients there is reduction in SHBG levels due to hyperinsulinemia, which results in increase in the amount of free circulating testosterones.

This insulin resistance may be due to defect in Tyrosine kinase receptor phosphorylation in Insulin receptor. In normal women tyrosine autophosphorylation occurs, which increases the insulin mediated metabolic changes within muscle and adipose tissue. But in PCOS women serine phosphorylation occurs, which inhibit this action and stimulate enzymatic activity in ovaries, which is responsible for production of androstenedione. Further in adipose tissue, insulin resistance results in increased hydrolysis of stored triglycerides and elevated circulating free fatty acid levels. Decrease glucose utilization in muscle and increased hepatic gluconeogenesis result in increased blood glucose concentration and a compensatory hyperinsulinemia. Thus, decrease in serum insulin levels would help in reducing the androgen levels. Hyperinsulinemia and insulin resistance are an important part of the pathophysiology of PCOS, but 25–50% of PCOS women does not demonstrate insulin resistance. So, it is not the primary pathogenetic factor in all PCOS women.

(d) Obesity and weight gain: The chance of developing PCOS rises in women with increasing obesity, along with the risk of hyperinsulinemia, ovulatory dysfunction, insulin resistance, metabolic syndrome, glucose intolerance and risk of cardiovascular disease. Obesity contributes to the pathogenesis in already affected women by aggravating the degree of hyperinsulinemia and insulin resistance.

6.5 Factors Drive to PCOS (Fig. 6.2)

1. Genetic predisposition—In PCOS a high level of familial clustering has been seen. In a study, it was found that daughters born to PCOS women has fivefold higher risk of PCOS as compared to those born to women without PCOS [8]. To elaborate the familial aggregation of PCOS, various gene have been associated studied. It includes genes are FSHB (follicle-stimulating hormone B polypeptide), AMH, FSHR (follicle stimulating hormone receptor), LHCGR (luteinizing hormone/choriogonadotropin receptor) and DENND1A (DENN domain containing 1A); and gene associated with metabolism such as INSR (insulin receptor) and THADA (thyroid adenoma-associated gene) [9].
2. Environmental factors—It includes follicular micro-environment, intrauterine environment of PCOS mother and lifestyle following birth. Evidence from vari-

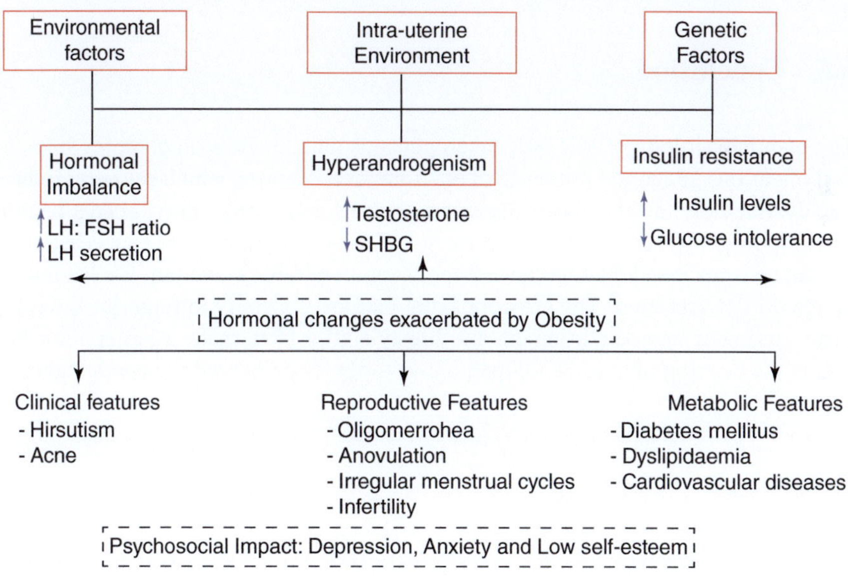

Fig. 6.2 Schematic illustration showing the risk factors like environmental, intra-uterine environment and genetic factors responsible for pathophysiology of PCOS and further development of clinical, metabolic and reproductive features. SHBG: Sex hormone binding globulin; LH: luteinizing hormone; FSH: Follicle stimulating hormone

ous studies suggest that prenatal exposure to increased androgen concentration may affect GnRH pulse programming, leading to increase pulse frequency and LH secretion. Hyperinsulinemia with high concentration of circulating AMH during pregnancy in mothers of PCOS also contribute to abnormal intrauterine environment. Unfavourable lifestyle which includes high glycaemic diet increases the risk of metabolic disease and PCOS. Exogenous toxin such as Endocrine disrupting chemicals or consumption of Advanced glycation end (AGE) products lead to development of PCOS. AGEs can form from smoking or high fat/protein diet, especially if this includes food items cooked in a low-moisture and high temperature.

Thus, hyperandrogenism from any cause, arising during adulthood (secondary to hyperinsulinemia, obesity), adolescence (nonclassical congenital adrenal hyperplasia, premature adrenarche) or in fetal life (due to maternal hyperandrogenism or classical CAH) causes abnormalities in the feedback control of pulsatile GnRH secretion, leading to increased LH secretion and further stimulating ovarian androgens production.

3. Another key feature of PCOS is follicular microenvironment pro-inflammatory state and low-grade systemic inflammation. It further exacerbates the pathogenesis along with ER stress and oxidative stress [10, 11]. Endoplasmic reticulum stress contributes to the pathophysiology of PCOS through multiple functional alterations in granulosa cells. ER stress accelerates interstitial fibrosis in the ovary and is associated with follicular arrest at the antral stage.

6.6 Conclusion

The pathophysiology of PCOS is heterogeneous and depends on complex interaction of various genes and influence of environmental factors, which cause reproductive dysfunction and metabolic disorders, with lifelong effect on women's health. Hyperandrogenism is the major feature in PCOS development. It is exacerbated by insulin resistance and dysfunctional hypothalamus-pituitary-ovarian axis leading to increased LH secretion. The environmental factors especially intrauterine environment, follicular microenvironment and lifestyle after birth make a larger contribution in the development of PCOS pathophysiology as compared to genetic factor.

References

1. Bozdag G, Mumusoglu S, Zengin D, Karabulut E, Yildiz BO. The prevalence and phenotypic features of polycystic ovary syndrome: a systematic review and meta-analysis. Hum Reprod. 2016;31:2841–55.
2. Azziz R, Carmina E, Dewailly D, Diamanti-Kandarakis E, Escobar-Morreale HF, Futterweit W, et al. Positions statement: criteria for defining polycystic ovary syndrome as a predominantly hyperandrogenic syndrome: an androgen excess society guideline. J Clin Endocrinol Metab. 2006;91:4237–45.

3. Kubota T. Update in polycystic ovary syndrome: new criteria of diagnosis and treatment in Japan. Reprod Med Biol. 2013;12:71–7.
4. Rotterdam ESHRE/ASRM-Sponsored PCOS Consensus Workshop Group. Revised 2003 consensus on diagnostic criteria and long-term health risks related to polycystic ovary syndrome (PCOS). Hum Reprod. 2004;19:41–7.
5. Clark NM, Podolski AJ, Brooks ED, Chizen DR, Pierson RA, Lehotay DC, Lujan ME. Prevalence of polycystic ovary syndrome phenotypes using updated criteria for polycystic ovarian morphology: an assessment of over 100 consecutive women self-reporting features of polycystic ovary syndrome. Reprod Sci. 2014;21:1034–43.
6. Guastella E, Longo RA, Carmina E. Clinical and endocrine characteristics of the main polycystic ovary syndrome phenotypes. Fertil Steril. 2010;94(6):2197–201.
7. Moghetti P, Tosi F, Bonin C, et al. Divergences in insulin resistance between the different phenotypes of the polycystic ovary syndrome. J Clin Endocrinol Metab. 2013;98(4):E628–37.
8. Coulam CB, Annegers JF, Kranz JS. Chronic anovulation syndrome and associated neoplasia. Obstet Gynecol. 1983;61(4):403–7.
9. Harada M. Pathophysiology of polycystic ovary syndrome revisited: current understanding and perspectives regarding future research. Reprod Med Biol. 2022;21:e12487.
10. Khan MJ, Ullah A, Basit S. Genetic basis of polycystic ovary syndrome (PCOS): current perspectives. Appl Clin Genet. 2019;12:249–60.
11. Taylor HS, Fritz MA, Pal L, Seli E. Speroff's clinical gynecologic endocrinology and infertility. 9th ed. Philadelphia, PA: Wolters Kluwer; 2020.

Chapter 7
PCOS Investigations and Clinical Implications

Sanjiv Kandhari

7.1 Definition of PCOS

Stein and Leventhal 1935 provided the first description of PCOS noting varying degrees of enlarged ovaries, obesity, hirsutism, and chronic anovulation. It is generally accepted that PCOS is not a specific endocrine disease but a syndrome represented by a collection of signs and symptoms [1–8].

- No one sign or symptom or test is diagnostic
- Thus, establishing diagnostic criteria for PCOS is both challenging and controversial
- In my view the primary advantage of diagnostic criteria is more important for researcher than **a** clinician, who understands the implications of the disease and treats them and may not require stringent criteria which a researcher requires for publication and conclusion

7.2 Diagnostic Criteria Changing with Time

- **1990—NICHD** diagnostic criteria were based upon traditional concepts requiring evidence of both **h**yperandrogenism, and or hyperandrogenemia, menstrual dysfunction (oligomenorrhea/amenorrhea)—**but no polycystic ovaries**
- **2003 ESHRE/ASRM Rotterdam criteria**—sought to include polycystic ovaries as evidence of ovarian dysfunction and included women having neither hyperandrogenism nor hirsutism, what it provided was an increased number of phenotypes and prevalence, **Three main phenotypes:**

S. Kandhari (✉)
Dr. Kandhari's Skin and Dental Clinic, New Delhi, India

R. Singh, N. Sharma (eds.), *A Guide to Hormonal Dermatology*,
https://doi.org/10.1007/978-981-99-7715-4_7

Table 7.1 A comparison of diagnostic criteria for polycystic ovary syndrome

1990 National Institute of Child Health and Human Development (NICHD) Guidelines Patient demonstrates both:
1. Clinical and/or biochemical signs of hyperandrogenism
2. Oligo- or chronic anovulation
Exclusion of other aetiologies of androgen excess and anovulatory infertility is necessary
2003 European Society for Human Reproduction and Embryology and American Society for Reproductive Medicine (ESHRE/ASRM or Rotterdam) Guidelines
Patient demonstrates two of three criteria:
1. Oligo- or chronic anovulation
2. Clinical and/or biochemical signs of hyperandrogenism
3. Polycystic ovaries
Exclusion of other aetiologies of androgen excess and anovulatory infertility is necessary.
2006 Androgen Excess Society (AES) Guideline:
Patient demonstrates both:
1. Hirsutism and/or hyperandrogenaemia
2. Oligo-anovulation and/or polycystic ovaries
Exclusion of other aetiologies of androgen excess and anovulatory infertility is necessary

1. Classic PCOS—Hyperandrogenism (HA), chronic oligo-anovulation, with or without PCOM
2. Ovulatory PCOS—HA, PCOM but ovulatory cycles
3. Chronic anovulation and polycystic ovaries, but no HA

- **2006 AE-PCOS society** allowed polycystic ovaries—which could be considered a sign of ovarian dysfunction but emphasized the importance of hyperandrogenism first including women with or without oligomenorrhoea or polycystic ovaries but excluding those having neither hyperandrogenism or hirsutism
- **All had exclusion of other androgen excess causes or related disorders in their criteria (Table 7.1)**

7.3 Diagnosis of PCOS: AACE/ACE2015

American Association of Clinical Endocrinologists (AACE) and the Androgen Excess and PCOS Society (AES)

Establishing hyperandrogenism	Establishing ovulatory dysfunction	Establishing PCOM
• **Androgens—Free testosterone**	• Cycle length is >35 days or less than 24 days	• **USG—Rotterdam guidelines—at least 12 follicles measuring** 2–9 mm in the whole ovary or by the finding of **increased ovarian size (>10 mL)**

Establishing hyperandrogenism	Establishing ovulatory dysfunction	Establishing PCOM
• By equilibrium dialysis techniques, if not available calculated T or **free androgen index(FAI) use:**	• Cycle length is −32 to 35 days or slightly irregular-**ovulation should be assessed**	• **New AES guidelines**—have increased the threshold count of **small ovarian follicles to 25 using 8 mm probe and a 4D u/s**
• Total testosterone × 100	• **Serum progesterone** during the midluteal phase	• **Anti-Müllerian hormone (AMH) value**
• ------------------------ SHBG		

AACE/AES PCOS Guidelines ENDOCRINE PRACTICE Vol 21 No. 11 November 2015 1291

7.4 What About Other Tests

- **Anti Mullerian hormone** (when u/s in doubt to diagnose PCOS)
- **SHBG** (Useful in calculating free testosterone)
- **Free androgen index** = (Total T/SHBG × 100)
- DHT (does not add value)
- Vit D3 (evidence lacking)
- **Serum progesterone:** helpful in checking ovulation in menstrual dysfunction at (mid luteal phase) 20–24 days, with Hyperandrogenism with eumenorrhea if progesterone is below 3–4 ng/mL then the cycle is deemed to be oligo-anovulatory
- Estradiol E2
- **TSH** (to r/o Non classical—PCOS)
- **Prolactin** (to r/o Non classical—PCOS)
- **17-OHP** (r/o NCCAH)
- **DHEAS** (lack of sensitivity/specificity-still useful in tumors)
- **Serum androstenedione** (value unclear)

7.5 Anti Mullerian Hormone (AMH)

- Women with PCOS have an increased number of small follicles in the pre antral and antral stage leading to a high AMH levels—which correlate well with AFC (antral follicle count)
- Elevated levels of AMH (>4.6 ng/dL) seen in normogonadotropic, normestrogenic, anovulatory patients compared with controls
- ↑AMH in PCOS whether obese or lean v/s women with no PCOS regardless of IR and adiposity status

- Non obese adolescents with PCOS had 1.49 times higher AMH levels v/s controls
- AMH levels are positively correlated with individual features of PCOS like ↑ LH, testosterone, mean ovarian volume, and number of ovarian follicles, and hyperandrogenism
- Levels of AMH help demarcate between women with classical PCOS and those with PCOS morphology alone (non classical PCOS)
- AMH also correlates with PCOS severity
- As a diagnostic marker AMH specificity is 92% and sensitivity 67%
- Where accurate U/S data not available AMH can be used instead of follicle count as a diagnostic criterion
- Useful to monitor therapeutic response to loss of weight, metformin and clomiphene citrate
- AMH values have marked changes in reproductive life span thus threshold values can change (biphasic effect in values with age)
- AMH assay values may change with the assay technique used

7.6 Serum 3ά-Diol G: As a Marker for Idiopathic Hirsutism (IH), PCOS with Hirsutism

- Since DHEAS and Androstenedione are the major precursors of 3ά-diol G the level of the conjugate either simply reflects adrenal and androgen biosynthesis
- Elevated levels simply reflect the presence of hirsutism regardless of the cause/ or excess production of DHEAS from any source
- Higher levels in IH—reflect only when all other causes of circulating androgens are normal but 20% of women with IH have normal 3ά-diol G, the levels of this hormone do not predict therapeutic response
- Thus, this test is NOT recommended in the evaluation of IH or any form of hirsutism, besides expensive and not available in most laboratories.

7.6.1 Alpha 3 Diol in Adult Acne

- A total of 60% of adult women with acne present increased levels of androgens
- And among those with normal levels and without menstrual dysfunctions,
- 50% show an increase in 3 alpha-diol G. Therefore, a pharmacological approach with anti-androgenic drugs for acne therapy in most of these patients is advisable.

Percentage of PCOS Ovarian Morphology Seen in Women With:

- Idiopathic hirsutism 92%
- Oligomenorrhoea 87%

- Congenital adrenal hyperplasia 82.3
- Amenorrhea 26%
- **Normal women with normal cycle 23%**
- **Women on contraceptives 18%**
- **PCOS 50 = 70%**

Polycystic ovaries do not establish and are not required for the diagnosis of PCOS as a sole criterion, as so many other conditions have the same morphology without other symptoms and signs of PCOS

7.6.2 Other Features of PCOS: Not Included in the Diagnostic Criteria

PCOS has other common features besides hyperandrogenism and ovulatory dysfunction that are not included in the diagnostic criteria

- Abnormal patterns of gonadotrophin secretion (LH/FSH)
- Insulin resistance (IR)-assessed by HOMA IR/Oral GTT—Can be used to asses both insulin sensitivity/resistance and glucose intolerance. The tests for insulin resistance (Table 7.2), In general 50–70% of PCOS have IR and hyperinsulinemia with metabolic syndrome
- Metabolic abnormalities such as dyslipidemias and
- Metabolic syndrome with increased cardiovascular risk

Table 7.2 Tests for insulin resistance

Name of test		
Fasting insulin **Post OGTT** **Fasting glucose/insulin**	Fasting >15 mU/mL (IR) >150 mU/mL (IR) <4.5 (IR)	
Hyper insulinemic **Euglycemic clamp**	**Gold standard**	
HOMA – IR **(Homeostatic model assessment)**	Glucose fasting × insulin mU/mL/22.5 **(>3.2–3.9 IR)**	
QUICKI **(Quantitative insulin sensitivity check index)**	1/log (insulin) + log glucose (F) **(>0.33-IR)**	
OGIS **(Oral glucose insulin sensitivity)**		
ORAL—GTT	**Glucose 2 h** Normal GTT <140 **Impaired 140–199** **DM >200**	**Insulin 2 h** Normal <80 to 100 **IR >80 to 100** Severe IR >300 mU/mL

Table 7.3 Exclusion of other androgen excess disorders as PCOS is a diagnosis of exclusion

Diagnosis	Method of exclusion
Non classical CAH -NCCAH	Follicular morning phase, levels of 17OHP, greater than 6.06nmol/l accounts for >90% of NCCAH, ACTH stimulation test further confirms the diagnosis. Definitive diagnosis requires a 17OHP concentration. >10NG/ML (30 NMOL/L). Either basally or after co-syntropin-stimulation, early onset hirsutism, family history-of CAH, high risk ethnicity
Androgen secreting tumor	Clinical S/S sudden onset hirsutism, high total serum testosterone >200 ng/dL
Severe IR syndrome	Clinical s/s, oral GTT (glucose and insulin)
Cushings syndrome	Clinical s/s, overnight dexa-suppression test
Idiopathic hirsutism	Menstrual history, serum progesterone (putative luteal phase), serum testosterone, SHBG low

7.6.3 Abnormal Gonadotrophin Secretion Measurements

How important is it for you to measure LH/ FSH ratios in PCOS patients in your practice?

LH/FSH no longer recommended:

There are differences in data supplied by different assays: (RIA with polyclonal antibodies, monoclonal antibody RIA, immunometric assays)

- **BMI affects levels**: Increased LH/FSH ratio are typical >2:1, more so in the lean than obese women with PCOS (where the basal levels are within normal range or LH/FSH ratio is not increased) and obesity is high with PCOS
- **Day of the cycle affects the level**
- Relationship of LH/FSH ratio in the pathogenesis of PCOS is unclear
- **Consequently, gonadotropin ratios are not a reliable marker as a diagnostic criterion they neither make, nor exclude, the diagnosis**

Exclusion of other androgen excess disorders as PCOS is a diagnosis of exclusion (Table 7.3).

Whereas all should be considered and excluded few actually warrant specific testing.

7.6.4 Summary and Key Points in Diagnosis of PCOS

- PCOS is not a specific endocrine disease but a syndrome represented by a collection of s/s and no one sign or symptom is diagnostic

- Diagnosis of PCOS is primarily based upon history and physical examination the major feature being hyperandrogenism and menstrual dysfunction
- Although present in most women with chronic hyper androgenic an ovulation, polycystic ovaries do not establish and are not required for the diagnosis of PCOS as the sole criteria.
- Gonadotropin levels or LH/FSH ratios are not a reliable criterion for the diagnosis of PCOS
- Knowing and understanding health implications of PCOS are far more important than assigning a diagnosis of PCOS

References

1. Azzizz R, et al. The Androgen Excess and PCOS Society criteria for the polycystic ovary syndrome: the complete task force report. Fertil Steril. 2009;91(2):456–88.
2. Conway G, et al. The polycystic ovary syndrome: a position statement from the European Society of Endocrinology. Eur J Endocrinol. 2014;171(4):P1–29.
3. Goodman NF, Cobin RH, et al. AACE/ACE disease state clinical review. Endocr Pract. 2015;21:1291.
4. Iliodromiti S, Kelsey TW, Anderson RA, Nelson SM. Can anti-Müllerian hormone predict the diagnosis of polycystic ovary syndrome? A systematic review and meta-analysis of extracted data. J Clin Endocrinol Metab. 2013;98:3332–40.
5. Lujan ME, Chizen DR, Pierson RA. Diagnostic criteria for polycystic ovary syndrome: pitfalls and controversies. J Obstet Gynaecol Can. 2008;30(8):671–9.
6. de Moura HHG, Costa DLM, Bagatin E, Sodré CT, Manela-Azulay M. Polycystic ovary syndrome: a dermatologic approach. An Bras Dermatol. 2011;86(1):111–9.
7. Housman E, Reynolds RV. Polycystic ovary syndrome: a review for dermatologists. Part I. Diagnosis and manifestations. J Am Acad Dermatol. 2014;71(5):847.e1–10.
8. Buzney E, Sheu J, Buzney C, Reynolds RV. Polycystic ovary syndrome: a review for dermatologists. Part II. Treatment. J Am Acad Dermatol. 2014;71:859.e1–15.

Chapter 8
PCOD-Management of ACNE

Apaopa Jemima Thekho and Rashmi Sarkar

8.1 Introduction

The most common endocrinological disorder among the reproductive age group is polycystic ovarian syndrome (PCOS) leading to various systemic dysfunction. It affects about 5–10% of the reproductive aged women [1]. Skin is a mirror of PCOS with considerable heterogeneity in the clinical findings and variation in same patient over time. 68% of the patients presented with cutaneous manifestations [2]. It alters the aesthetic qualities of a woman by features of hyperandrogenism which are clinically manifested as hirsutism, acne, seborrhoea, female pattern alopecia and acanthosis nigricans. Hirsutism and acanthosis nigricans are the most reliable cutaneous markers of PCOS. Though common, acne and androgenetic alopecia are unreliable markers of hyperandrogenism.

Acne vulgaris has a polymorphic nature, easy to diagnose, however difficult to evaluate its severity. Acne is seen in around 20–40% of PCOS women in different studies [3]. They exhibited facial acne lesions, as well as on neck, chest and upper back. It should be differentiated from acne vulgaris as

- usually distributed in the lower half of face and jaw-line (V-distribution).
- menstrual flare is common.
- often fails to respond to the conventional therapy
- other features of hyperandrogenism.

Acne has various measurement scales which are used based on the course of the disease. They include clinical examination and photographic documentation (Table 8.1).

A. J. Thekho · R. Sarkar (✉)
Department of Dermatology and Venereology, Lady Hardinge Medical College and Kalawati Saran Children Hospital, New Delhi, India

R. Singh, N. Sharma (eds.), *A Guide to Hormonal Dermatology*,
https://doi.org/10.1007/978-981-99-7715-4_8

Table 8.1 Grading of acne severity: Based on predominant lesions (Pillsbury, Shelley and Kligman)

Grade I	Comedones, occasional papules
Grade II	Comedones, many papules, few pustules
Grade III	Predominant pustules, nodules, abscesses
Grade IV	Mainly cysts, abscesses, scars

Table 8.2 Diagnostic Criteria for PCOS

1. Hyperandrogenism
2. Ovulatory dysfunction
3. Polycystic ovarian morphology (>12 follicles, 2–9 mm in diameter with volume of >10 mL in at least one ovary)

Table 8.3 Investigations in PCOS

1. Hormonal profile-Total testosterone, androstenedione, prolactin, 17-OH progesterone, DHEAS, LH/FSH ratio
2. Serum fasting insulin
3. Ultrasonography of pelvis
4. Metabolic profile-lipid profile, blood sugar, fasting insulin
5. Others-TSH, AMH

The diagnosis of PCOS is currently established by the 2003 Rotterdam Consensus criteria defined by the presence of two of three of the following criteria (Table 8.2).

As there is no single test to make the diagnosis, the final diagnosis is based on clinical features, physical findings and few laboratory investigations summarised in Table 8.3.

Lab Investigations: Baseline screening for laboratory hyperandrogeniemia should be done. It can be assessed by measuring common androgens, testosterone (total or free), androstenedione, DHEA, and DHEA-metabolite DHEAS. It is recommended to measure free testosterone rather than total one because SHBG is reduced in hyperandrogenism which is the main determinant of bioavailable testosterone [4]. Test should be performed early in the morning and preferable between day fourth and day tenth of menstrual cycle ideally. However elevated level of testosterone is not the sole criterion to diagnose hyperandrogenism as 20–40% of women with PCOS, androgen levels are in normal range and total testosterone levels are variable [5].

Even DHEA has limited diagnostic value, but DHEAS can be measured to exclude adrenal cause. Other biochemical tests are Thyroid stimulating hormone, prolactin, 17 hydroxy progesterone, dexamethasone suppression test, and 24 h urinary cortisol which are done to exclude other causes which also mimic PCOS.

There is increased secretion of LH, increased GnRH/LH pulsatility, and normal FSH. The raised LH/FSH ratio is considered a marker of PCOS.

Insulin resistance and raised insulin levels may be seen in a majority of patients with PCOS. The standard 2 h oral glucose tolerance test (OGTT) is considered to be the best way to assess both insulin and glucose yield [5]. OGTT should be done only when fasting blood glucose level is <110 mg/dL (normal) or impaired (110–125 mg/

dL). A ratio of fasting glucose to fasting insulin is a simple and effective alternative. A ratio of less than 7 is highly suggestive of a hyperinsulenemic state.

Anti mullerian hormone is expressed by the granulosa cells of the ovarian follicles. The assay help in assessing the follicular count and it is significantly higher in women with polycystic ovarian syndrome.

The ovarian morphology is better depicted on trans-vaginal ultrasound examination.

Trans-abdominal ultrasound examination is preferred in adolescents and mandatory in unmarried women. It is best performed within few days of menstrual bleeding to avoid any confusion of the dominant follicle. The USG classically shows multiple subcentimeter cysts (>12, 2–9 mm) within the ovaries. The "string of pearls" appearance (peripheral arrangement of the follicles surrounding a central echogenic stroma), though characteristic, is not a requirement for diagnosis. The other ultrasonographic feature is that the volume of the ovaries should be each more than 10 cc.

Metabolic derangements are common in these patients, hence blood sugars, lipid profile and BMI calculation and waist circumference should be done.

8.2 Management

8.2.1 Non-hormonal Therapy

1. Life-style modifications includes low-calorie diet, regular exercise and weight loss is recommended as the first-line management [6]. The reduction of total body weight by 5% reduces the insulin resistance and testosterone levels.
2. Non hormonal therapy for acne

   Treatment recommendations is standard acne therapy according to European guidelines [7].

   (a) Comedonal acne

   - First line-topical retinoids (adapalene>tretinoin)
   - Second line-Benzoyl peroxide(BPO) or azelaic acid

   (b) Mild to moderate papulopustular acne

   - First line-BPO + adapalene or BPO + clindamycin
   - Second line-BPO or azelaic acid or systemic antibiotic + adapalene
   - Third line-Isotretinoin or tretinoin+ topical erythromycin
     - Systemic antibiotics + BPO

   (c) Severe papulopustular/mild nodular acne

   - First line-systemic isotretinoin
   - Second line-systemic antibiotics + adapalene; systemic antibiotics + azelaic acid; systemic antibiotics+BPO+ adapalene

   (d) Third line-Hormonal antiandrogens+ topical treatment/systemic antibiotics

(e) Severe nodular acne and conglobata acne

- First line-systemic isotretinoin
- Second line-systemic antibiotics + azelaic acid/BPO/BPO+ adapalene (f.c.)

8.2.2 *Oral Isotretinoin*

It remains the most clinically effective therapy for acne. It suppresses sebum secretion, inhibits bacterial proliferation, normalizes keratinization with anti-inflammatory activity. A dose of 0.5–1.0 mg/kg/day is recommended.

The most common side-effects inclues dryness of skin and mucosa, deranged metabolic profile and liver enzymes. In women of reproductive age group, it is advised to avoid pregnancy during and 1 month after therapy.

8.2.3 *Oral Antibiotics*

Oral antibiotics are recommended as second-line therapy for short-term management and as an adjunctive therapy when hormonal therapy are inadequate [9]. They are used for inflammatory acne because of their antibiotic and anti-inflammatory effects. The tetracyclines are the antibiotics of choice most commonly used agents includes doxycycline, minocycline and sarecycline. Other antimicrobial agents used are macrolides (erythromycin, clindamycin or azithromycin), trimethoprim are used when tetracyclines are not tolerated or containdicated [10].

8.2.3.1 Hormonal Therapy

Hormonal therapy aims to suppress androgen production from ovaries, adrenals and pituitary and it also inhibits the ARs on sebaceous gland however it is not indicated as a monotherapy [11]. The indications of hormonal treatment include

1. Acne not responding to conventional treatment
2. Severe flare-ups before menstruation
3. When contraception or menstrual control is desirable
4. Polycystic ovary syndrome
5. When isotretinoin is contraindicated or unavailable

The European guidelines on acne therapy recommend hormonal treatment along with topical or systemic antibiotics in severe pustular and moderate nodulocystic acne cases as an alternative to starting therapy with isotretinoin. In severe type of acne, antibiotics along with hormonal treatment are recommended. Hormonal therapy is effective in acne despite elevated androgen levels or not. A course of 3 months is often necessary before experiencing benefit from the treatment [12]. Clascoterone, a topical androgen receptor inhibitor has been approved by the FDA in a twice daily application, 1% cream formulation in patients aged 12 years and older.

8.2.4 *Combined Oral Contraceptives*

They are recommended as first-line therapy unless contraindicated. Ethinyl estradiol is the most common estrogen component which suppress gonadotropin secretion and ovarian steroid synthesis, with reduced level of free circulating testosterone and serum androgens. Progestins such as desogestrel, drosperinone, cyproterone acetate has anti-androgenic activity is potentially effective in acne. Drospirenone is the only progestin approved by the Food and Drug Administration (FDA), which blocks the AR and is truly antiandrogenic, even without the addition of estrogen [11].

It is initiated from day 1 of the menstrual cycle and for 21 days on/7 days off fashion, for five to six cycles.

Based on WHO recommendations, the use of COCs is absolutely contraindicated in pregnancy, history of thromboembolism, liver disease, smokers, aged ≥35 years, while relative contraindications include breastfeeding, hypertension, migraine, and existing malignancies. Moreover, certain conditions might be worsened by contraceptives such as insulin resistance and is contraindicated in diabetic patients, clotting disorders, and in patients with increased risk of breast cancer.

8.2.5 *Spironolactone*

It is an aldosterone antagonist with antiandrogenic properties. It inhibits steroidogenesis and 5-α reductase-activity. The usual dosage for the treatment of acne is 50–100 mg/day. Spironolactone maybe used in conjunction with oral contraceptives.

Side-effects with this recommended dose are minimal. However, women should be advised to be on birth control while on this medication to avoid feminization of male fetus in an unplanned pregnancy and to consume high potassium containing food items.

8.2.6 *Androgen Receptor Blockers*

8.2.6.1 Cyproterone Acetate

CPA is an antiandrogen which suppress sebum. It is very effective when used as a monotherapy showing significant improvement with doses of 50–100 mg/d from days 1–10 of the menstrual cycle.

Despite its monotherapy high rates of clearance, it is usually combined with estrogen in the oral contraceptive pill (OCP) in doses of 2 mg with 35 μg of ethinyl estradiol.

8.2.6.2 Flutamide

Flutamide is approved for the treatment of cancer prostate. It is a non-steroidal androgen receptor antagonist and is effective to treat acne, androgenetic alopecia, and hirsutism. It is used in low doses ranging from as low as 62.5–125 mg/day. The combination of OCPs and flutamide was more efficacious than flutamide alone [8].

Side effects include breast tenderness, gastrointestinal upset, insomnia and fatigue.

8.2.6.3 Insulin-Sensitizing Agents

These agents are used to decrease androgen production by reducing the hyperinsulinemia. Metformin is used for acne in association with other evidence of hyperinsulinemia. Treatment is started with a dose of 500 mg and up to 2000 mg/d.

Most side effects are dose dependent and include nausea and vomiting, hypoglycemia.

8.2.6.4 Psychological Support

PCOS women has an increased risk of developing psychological and behavioral changes due to impaired feminine identity, obesity and long term morbidity hence timely counselling and adequate intervention should be offered.

References

1. Patel S. Polycystic ovary syndrome (PCOS), an inflammatory, systemic, lifestyle endocrinopathy. J Steroid Biochem Mol Biol. 2018;182:27–36. https://doi.org/10.1016/j.jsbmb.2018.04.008.
2. Aljefri YE, et al. Cutaneous manifestations and hormonal changes among polycystic ovary syndrome patients at a tertiary care center. Cureus. 2021;13(12):e20593.

3. Gainder S, Sharma B. Update on management of polycystic ovarian syndrome for dermatologists. Indian Dermatol Online J. 2019;10(2):97.
4. Norman RJ, Dewailly D, Legro RS, Hickey TE. Polycystic ovary syndrome. Lancet. 2007;370(9588):685–97.
5. Azziz R, et al. The androgen excess and PCOS society criteria for the polycystic ovary syndrome: the complete task force report. Fertil Steril. 2009;91(2):456–88.
6. Teede HJ, et al. Translation and implementation of the Australian-led PCOS guideline: clinical summary and translation resources from the international evidence-based guideline for the assessment and management of polycystic ovary syndrome. Med J Aust. 2018;209:S3–8.
7. Nast A, Dreno B, Bettoli V, Degitz K, Erdmann R, Finlay AY, Ganceviciene R, Haedersdal M, Layton A, López-Estebaranz JL, Ochsendorf F. European evidence-based (S3) guidelines for the treatment of acne. J Eur Acad Dermatol Venereol. 2012;26:1–29.
8. Chuan SS, Chang RJ. Polycystic ovary syndrome and acne. Skin Therapy Lett. 2010;15(10):1–4.
9. Buzney E, Sheu J, Buzney C, Reynolds RV. Polycystic ovary syndrome: a review for dermatologists: part II treatment. J Am Acad Dermatol. 2014;71(5):859–e1.
10. Tan AU, Schlosser BJ, Paller AS. A review of diagnosis and treatment of acne in adult female patients. Int J Women's Dermatol. 2018;4(2):56–71.
11. Elsaie ML. Hormonal treatment of acne vulgaris: an update. Clin Cosmet Investig Dermatol. 2016;9:241.
12. Harper JC. Use of oral contraceptives for management of acne vulgaris: practical considerations in real world practice. Dermatol Clin. 2016;34(2):159–65.

Chapter 9
Management of Pigmentation in Polycystic Ovary Syndrome

Rashmi Shetty and Meera Govindaraju

9.1 Introduction

Polycystic ovary syndrome (PCOS) affects 6–10% women of fertile age group. While PCOS presents with many cutaneous manifestations, this chapter is dedicated to pigmentary changes such as acanthosis nigricans, acrochordons, DPN, seborrheic dermatitis, hidradenitis suppurativa, post acne PIH and melasma. Recent study shows that PCOS is associated with obesity, insulin resistance (IR), diabetes mellitus [1] and other metabolic syndromes leading to various presentations of hyperpigmentation and excess androgen. Pigmentation is often an important cosmetic concern that affects the overall well-being of a PCOS patient and therefore the need to address and correct the same to the best possible extent.

Alongside clinical assessment and history taking, a set of laboratory work helps in clinching the diagnosis as well as choosing the right treatment process (Table 9.1, Fig. 9.1) .

R. Shetty (✉)
RA Clinics, Mumbai/Hyderabad, India
e-mail: Rashmi@drrashmishetty.com

M. Govindaraju
Chennai, India

R. Singh, N. Sharma (eds.), *A Guide to Hormonal Dermatology*,
https://doi.org/10.1007/978-981-99-7715-4_9

Table 9.1 Laboratory Bloodwork for Pigmentation in PCOS

• Fasting and post prandial glucose
• Fasting and post prandial insulin levels
• C- Reactive protein
• Hb1Ac
• HOMA index
• Serum prolactin
• Thyroid levels[a]
• ACTH[a]
• 8 am Serum cortisol[a]
• Vitamin b12[a]

[a]To exclude other contributory factors towards pigmentary change

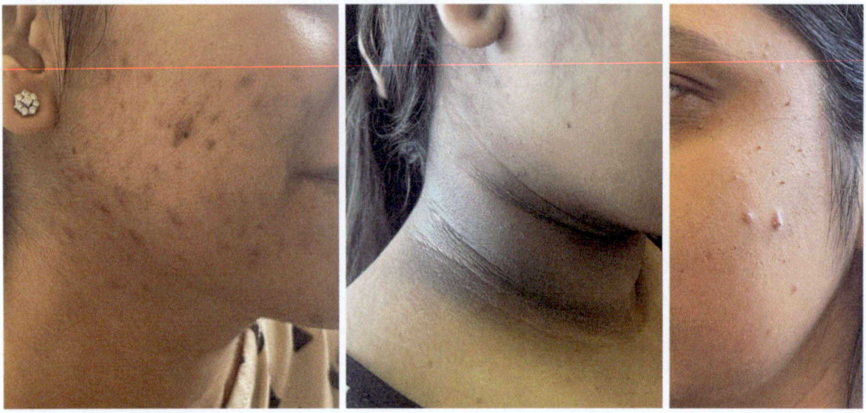

Fig. 9.1 Acne induced post inflammatory hyperpigmentation, Pseudo acanthosis nigricans(neck), DPN/ Acrochordans (Left to Right)

9.2 Acanthosis Nigricans

Acanthosis Nigricans (AN) is a cutaneous marker for hyperinsulinemia in PCOS. Most cases are linked to obesity and insulin resistance [2, 3]. AN present with velvety brown, thickened plaques, and accentuated skin markings. Usually localized to the nape and sides of the neck. Other common sites of involvement are axillae, groin, anogenital and inframammary region. Facial acanthosis [4] which commonly affects the forehead and temples followed by zygomatic and mandibular areas is easily missed which also needs equal attention. Extensive presentation of AN should alert clinicians on malignancy as in involvement of mucous membranes and mucocutaneous junctions [5].

Histology shows papillomatosis, hyperkeratosis, and slight acanthosis with minimal or no hyperpigmentation in the basal layer [6, 7]. Clinically observed hyperpigmentation is due to hyperkeratosis and not secondary melanin deposition as seen in other pigmentary disorders.

9.2.1 *Treatment*

As obesity is an important cause for insulin resistance, lifestyle counselling plays a pivotal role. Regular cardiovascular exercises, stress relieving activities like meditation and yoga along with dietary changes such as avoiding high glycaemic indexed food and calorie restriction. Also, time of food intake like early dinners, small frequent meals and intermittent fasting are types of dietary habits that have gained popularity in recent times and rightly so.

9.2.1.1 General Counselling

Patients need to be counselled against usage of harsh chemicals, or DIY home based treatments like flour-based scrubs & lemon juice, which may worsen the existing condition.

9.2.1.2 Topical Medications

Topical treatments are aimed at reducing the hyperkeratosis and those that reduce the hyperpigmentation.

Topical treatments aimed at Hyperkeratosis.

1. Surface keratolytic such as Salicylic acid, urea, and ammonium lactate.
2. Topical retinoids work by causing alteration in epidermal keratinization [8]. Calcipotriene, a vitamin D analog inhibits keratinocyte proliferation and promotes differentiation by increasing keratinocyte intracellular calcium and Cyclic GMP levels [9]. Calcipotriol downregulates the number of keratinocytes [10] resulting in reducing the cutaneous effects of AN.

Topical treatments aimed at Hyperpigmentation.

1. Skin lightening agents, which work at various pathways of melanin production and transfer, such as Azelaic acid, kojic acid, arbutin, hydroquinone and AHAs.

9.2.1.3 Systemic Medications

Oral retinoids have proven beneficial in few cases. They act by normalizing the epidermal growth and differentiation [9, 11]. Additionally, correction of hyperinsulinemia with drugs like metformin [12] which improves the insulin sensitivity, thaizolidinediones [13], sitagliptin—increases the insulin secretion) and octreotide are beneficial.

Fish oils containing omega 3 fatty acids, oral anti-inflammatory drugs which contain superoxide dismutase, alpha lipoic acid, selenium, and supplements which have antioxidants like polypodium leucotomos, carotenoids and chromium picolinate have been found useful as adjuvant therapy.

9.2.1.4 In-Clinic Treatment

- Chemical Peels like salicylic acid, phenol peel, mandelic acid, lactic acid, kojic acid and combination peels like Jessners peel, as well as stay on peels like retinol peels are used, depending on what down time is acceptable to the patient. However, multiple sittings, along with lifestyle modification and medications are key in achieving good results.
- Long pulse alexandrite [14]laser have been found to give more promising results in AN.

9.3 Hyperprolactinemia

Excess prolactin level is commonly reported in PCOS patients. Higher prolactin levels can cause redness of the skin and is associated with insulin resistance. This resistant state may be the result of serum free fatty acids (FFA) [15] levels, by a down-regulation of number of insulin receptors or post-binding defect in insulin action or more.

9.3.1 Treatment

A treatment course that includes correcting the inflammatory component with topical antioxidants and anti-inflammatory applications, and repairing the skin barrier with moisturisers and sunscreen will add to the overall result.

9.3.1.1 Systemic Medications

Genes involved in vitamin D metabolism have been suggested as candidate genes for the susceptibility to PCOS. Non obese insulin resistant PCOS patients with excess prolactin [16] levels have reported reduced vitamin D levels. Therefore, correction of vitamin D deficiencies becomes vital. Oral cabergoline can be given in collaboration with an endocrinologist.

Oral anti-inflammatory agents such as N Acetyl cysteine, Resveratrol, super oxide dismutase, quercetin, rosemary, and vitamin C act as good supportive therapies.

9.3.1.2 Pro Tip

Prokinetics [17] increase prolactin levels. As PCOS patients may have eating disorders while battling the obesity, frequent use of prokinetics which increases the prolactin levels needs to be kept under radar.

9.4 Seborrheic Dermatitis

Excess androgens as in PCOS stimulates excess production of sebaceous secretion. Seborrheic dermatitis is an inflammatory disorder presenting greasy looking, yellowish scales with erythema in the seborrheic zones of the body. In PCOS patients, insulin resistance and increased IGF-1 and DHT could also cause pigmentation in seborrheic skin, which includes the transverse nasal groove, crease of the alae of nose and the supramental crease. Inflammatory aggregates [18] in the seborrheic areas disrupt the epidermal barrier causing an immune response to Malassezia furfur yeasts. Temples, forehead and T zone are the other areas which can show pigmentation.

9.4.1 Treatment

9.4.1.1 General Instruction

Taking care of excess seborrhoea of both scalp and facial skin is of primary importance during the treatment.

9.4.1.2 Topicals

Skin care regimes with AHA, BHA and PHAs containing formulations in the form of facewash, toner, serums or face creams and scalp care with BHAs, and antifungal shampoos help in controlling the seborrhoea of the face and scalp, respectively.

Tea tree oil, plant derived bakuchiol, topical retinoids and topical antifungals are established ingredients contributes to treatment outcome.

9.4.1.3 Systemic Medications

Oral low dose of isotretinoin and systemic antifungals help in reducing the local colonization of M.furfur.

9.4.1.4 In-Clinic Treatment

In-clinic treatments include Micro needling with radiofrequency which reduces the gland hypersecretion. Additionally, HydraFacial's and BHA based peels assist in outcome achievement.

9.5 Post Acne PIH

Severe and long-standing acne not responding to treatment could be one of the presenting symptoms of a PCOS patient at a dermatologist's clinic. This therefore leads to scarring and pigmentation, which can be severe, traumatic, and challenging to treat. Severe cystic acne, acne fulminans, usage of home-based DIYs or simply due to delay in seeking treatment can present with post acne PIH and scarring of the skin. Patients with acne excoriee tend to exhibit increased scarring and pigmentation post and during active acne. Severe scarring due to hidradenitis suppurativa (HS) which could be hypertrophic pigmented scar as well as severe hyperpigmentation is yet another condition associated with PCOS.

Progress of acne associated with PCOS does not exhibit a linear and fixed pattern. Therefore, PIH is not only observed after acne is treated but could be a part of the active lesions during the initial treatment phase. Initial stages of acne present with inflammation or as erythematous spots slowly progressing to brownish black or black colour discolouration according to the skin type of the patient.

9.5.1 Treatment

A detailed counselling session is essential in treating PIH, especially among PCOS patients. Prescribing the patient, a skin care regime which aims at making the skin less irritable or less sensitive and facilitates repairing of the skin barrier can help prevent the PIH. Additionally, barrier protection with lifestyle modifications such avoiding excessive sun exposure, avoiding aggressive DIY skin treatments at home, blue light protection, regular usage of sunscreen and moisturisers help in reducing the chances of PIH.

9.5.1.1 General Instructions

Patient should be counselled against popping the pimples and picking on it. Giving spot correctors and SOS measures which are medically appropriate will reduce the anxiety hence reducing the need to resort to home based DIY measures which could lead to further irritation of the already inflamed skin.

9.5.1.2 Topical Therapy

- Topical retinoids—Normalizing follicular desquamation.
- Tyrosinase inhibitors—Azelaic acid, kojic acid, quercetin also helps in reducing the pigmentation.
- Skin lightening agents—Hydroquinone, tranexamic acid, niacinamide, ascorbic acid, arbutin, liquorice extract are also used.

9.5.1.3 Oral Drugs

Oral sunscreens like polypodium leucotomos, along with oral anti-inflammatory agents such as milk thistle, rosemary, ginger, and curcumin help in reducing the inflammatory component, thereby reducing the PIH. Antioxidants with good UV protection properties like N Acetyl cysteine, resveratrol, quercetin and green tea polyphenols are other oral treatment options available. Oral vitamins like Vit b12, Vitamin C and K have been are useful adjuvant treatment methods.

9.5.1.4 Pro Tip

During history taking, if patients reveal tendency to PIH elsewhere in the body, it is suggested to avoid antibiotics which increases photosensitivity and therefore PIH, such as doxycycline, minocycline, and oral retinoids. PCOS patients require repeated and long-term antibiotics. Hence, these antibiotics, if required, are better given as short courses.

9.5.1.5 In-Clinic Treatments

Chemical peels, lasers and energy-based devices are the inclinic treatment options available for post acne PIH. In clinic treatments are as follows.

Skin lightening peels

- Lactic acid
- Mandelic acid
- Glycolic peel 35–50%
- Ferulic acid peel
- Miami peel—salicylic acid, green tea extract, ascorbic acid, antioxidant
- Black peel—Sulfur, acetic acid and SA
- Retinol
- Combination or sequential peels—SA, Mandelic acid or TCA for ice-pick scars

9.5.1.6 Lasers and EBD

Lasers & Energy Based Devices

- Q switch nano Nd:YAG (532,1064 nm)
- Q switch Ruby laser (694 nm)
- Alexandrite (755 nm)
- Pulsed dye laser
- Intense pulsed light
- Intralesional steroids/5FU are more useful with hypertrophic pigmented scar of HS.

9.6 DPN/Acrochordans

Dermatosis Papulosa nigra and acrochordans otherwise called as fibroepithelial polyps or skin tags is found to be commonly associated with type 2 diabetes mellitus, obesity, and insulin resistance [19–23]. DPN are benign epidermal growth seen as hyperpigmented spots during early stages. Acrochordons are loose oedematous tissue growth with a fibrovascular core and chronic inflammation. Usually seen in intertriginous areas like axilla, groin, and neck. Size ranges from 2 to 5 mm and soft velvety outgrowths. During early stages it can present as hyperpigmentation which slowly progresses to become polyps in those with predisposing factors.

Treatment includes snipping off the lesion with scissors, light electro curettage or light electrodessication and radiofrequency ablation. Ablative co2 lasers are used when they are of bigger size.

9.7 Melasma

Melasma is an acquired skin disorder presenting with hyper melanosis/ hyperpigmentation predominantly over the sun exposed area, though rarely can involve neck and forearms. HP: The melanocytes were larger, more dendritic and showed increased melanogenesis there was no increase in number of melanocyte [24].

Increased incidence in women of childbearing age suggests that female hormones have a role to play.

Certain melasma patients showed increased luteinizing hormone and reduced oestradiol levels which is suggestive of mild ovarian dysfunction [25]. Likewise, Hassan and Farhana et al. also reported increased levels of LH and lower levels of prolactin [26]. Higher rate of enlarged, multicystic ovaries and hirsutism were seen in melasma patients [27]. These studies suggest incidence of melasma in the background of a hormonal cause suggesting a link between PCOS and melasma.

9.7.1 General Instructions

9.7.2 Topical Treatment

Traditional depigmenting agents hydroquinone, kojic acid, arbutin, azelaic acid and other triple combinations like kligmans formula {5% HQ, 0.1% tretinoin and 0.1% dexamethasone} or modified kligmans formula {4%HQ, 0.05% tretinoin and 1% hydrocortisone acetate} are being used with good results.

Newer topical skin lightening agents that can be used for all the above pigmentary conditions (Tables 9.2 and 9.3).

In general, antioxidants which are substances that scavenges the free radicals produced during oxidative stress, anti-inflammatory with UV protective properties, oral photoprotectors are beneficial for an inflammatory disorder like PCOS.

Table 9.2 Newer skin lightening agents

Tranexamic acid	Inhibits plasmin
5% cysteamine cream	Reduces melanogenic enzymes in melanogenesis pathway
Zinc sulfate	Anti oxidant and photoprotective
Rucinol 1%	Tyrosinase inhibitor
Mulberry extract	Scavenges ROS
Flutamide 1%	Blocks endo and exogenous testosterone by binding to androgen receptors
Methimazole [28]	Peroxidase inhibitor that blocks melanin synthesis
Dioic acid 1%	Reduces tyrosinase mRNA by binding to peroxisome proliferator-activated receptor gamma
N acetyl glucosamine	Reduces melanin production and decreases melanosome transport inside the cell
Lignin peroxidase [29]	Eumelanin degradation in epidermis along with activator component h_2o_2
Niacinamide 4%	Inhibits melanosome transfer

Table 9.3 Supportive Systemic Medications in the treatment of hyperpigmentation

- Tranexamic acid
- Procyanidins/ Pycnogenol
- Polypodium leucotomos
- Glutathione
- Vitamin C
- Melatonin

Table 9.4 Chemical peels

• Glycolic acids 50–70%
• TCA 10–30%
• Jessner's peel
• Modified tretinoin peels
• Amino acid peels
• Lipohydroxy acid peels—a derivative of salicylic acid

Table 9.5 Various lasers used in the treatment of hyperpigmentation

• Q switch Nd:YAG laser
• Fractionated Er:YAG
• Fractional Erbium glass laser
• Fractional Co_2 laser
• Fractional thulium laser—longer remission rate
• Copper bromide laser, q-switched alexandrite, q-switched ruby and fractioned IPL [31, 32]

9.7.3 *In-Clinic Treatment*

Mesotherapy with microinjection [30] of tranexamic acid have proven beneficial in few cases. Additionally, meso injection of vitamin C and glutathione are also found to be useful (Table 9.4).

Above mentioned peels along with topical skin lightening agents have shown positive results. Refer Table 9.2.

9.7.4 *Lasers and EBD*

Q-switched Nd:YAG laser as monotherapy is shown to be more efficacious than IPL or TCA peels. However Relapse rate could be more common with combination therapies of Nd:YAG and IPL and aggressive energy settings (Table 9.5).

9.8 Laser Induced Hyperpigmentation

Lasers are advocated for PCOS patients presenting with hirsutism, pigmentation and acne. Unlike treating patients with idiopathic hirsutism, treating excessive hair growth in PCOS patients is challenging as it requires multiple sessions for reduction in hair growth. Diode, long pulsed Neodymium:YAG laser, long pulsed alexandrite lasers(755 nm), ruby laser(694 nm) and intense pulsed light therapy are the various lasers used in the treatment of hair reduction in hirsutism. Treatment with various lasers can result in undue pigmentation on dark skin.

Adverse effect profile is generally higher with ruby lasers and IPL especially when operated by inexperienced hands. Potential complications from IPL hair removal with excessive energy or improper technique include iatrogenic hyperpigmentation, hypopigmentation, folliculitis, and paradoxical hypertrichosis [33].

Pre-existing conditions of pigmentation and inflammation by itself in PCOS patients pose a great challenge to the clinician in choosing the right energy levels/fluences, spot size, pulse width and the skin types is of primal importance in achieving the maximum desirable results without adverse effects.

9.8.1 Treatment

9.8.1.1 General Care

Pre and post cooling of the area to be treated is of utmost importance as it reduces the chances of hyperpigmentation that might happen due to higher fluences used for thicker hair especially in darker skin. Post procedure topical steroids helps in minimizing the risk of PIH. Strict sun protection with sunscreen after the laser hair reduction procedure is also necessary in reducing the risk of pigmentation.

9.8.1.2 Topical Therapy

Skin lightening agents like kojic acid, glycolic acid, arbutin and vitamin C are used. Application of topical steroids for short durations are helpful in the case of severe conditions.

9.8.1.3 Oral Treatment

Oral antioxidants and oral sunscreens help in reducing the pigmentation.

9.8.1.4 In-Clinic Treatment

As mentioned earlier, various skin lightening peels repeated at frequent intervals in combination with lasers spaced accordingly helps in reducing the hyperpigmentation. Q switch nano sec Nd:YAG and pico lasers are helpful in reducing the iatrogenic hyperpigmentation .

9.9 Conclusion

Hyperpigmentation in PCOS is a distressing condition. It is vital to find the underlying cause as well as it is trigger factors. Initiation of early treatment and correcting the underlying cause helps in reducing the pigmentary condition to a great extent thus relieving the cosmetic concern of a systemic disorder like PCOS.

References

1. Lee H, Oh JY, Sung YA, Chung H, Cho WY. The prevalence and risk factors for glucose intolerance in young Korean women with polycystic ovary syndrome. Endocrine. 2009;36:326–32.
2. Hud JA Jr, Cohen JB, Wagner JM, et al. Prevalence and significance of acanthosis nigricans in an adult obese population. Arch Dermatol. 1992;128(7):941–4.
3. Brockow K, Steinkraus V, Rinninger F, et al. Acanthosis nigricans : a marker for early sign of hyperinsulinemia. Pediatr Dermatol. 1995;12(4):323–6.
4. Anon. Indian J Dermatol. 2017;62(6):591–7. https://doi.org/10.4103/ijd.IJD_545_17.
5. Schwartz RA. Acanthosis nigricans. J Am Acad Dermatol. 1994;31(1):1–19: quiz 20-22.
6. McKee PH, Calonje E, Granter SR. Pathology of the skin. 3rd ed. Philadelphia: Elsevier Mosby; 2005.
7. Hermanns-Le T, Scheen A, Pierard GE. Acanthosis nigricans associated with insulin resistance: pathophysiology and management. Am J Clin Dermatol. 2004;5(3):199–203.
8. Schwartz RA. Efficacy of topical 0.1% adapalene gel for use in the treatment of childhood acanthosis nigricans: a pilot study. Dermatol Ther. 2015;28(4):266.
9. Phiske MM. An approach to acanthosis nigricans. Indian Dermatol Online J. 2014;5(3):239–49.
10. Romo A, Benavides S. Treatment options in insulin resistance obesity-related acanthosis nigricans. Ann Pharmacother. 2008;42(7–8):1090–4.
11. Jeong K-H, Oh S-J, Chon S, Lee MH. Generalized acanthosis nigricans related to type B insulin resistance syndrome: a case report. Cutis. 2010;86:299–302.
12. Tankova T, Koev D, Dakovska L, Kirilov G. Therapeutic approach in insulin resistance with acanthosis nigricans. Int J Clin Pract. 2002;56(8):578–81.
13. Atabek ME, Pirgon O. Use of metformin in obese adolescents with hyperinsulinemia: a 6-month, randomized, double-blind, placebo-controlled clinical trial. J Pediatr Endocrinol Metab. 2008;21(4):339–48.
14. Rosenbach A, Ram R. Treatment of acanthosis nigricans of the axillae using a long-pulsed (5-msec) alexandrite laser. Dermatologic Surg. 2004;30(8):1158–60.
15. Tuzcu A, Bahceci M, Dursun M, Turgut C, Bahceci SJ. Endocrinol Invest. 2003;26(4):341–6. https://doi.org/10.1007/BF03345182.
16. Anon. J Endocrinol Invest. 2003;26(7):655–9. https://doi.org/10.1007/BF03347025.
17. Anon. Pharmacological causes of hyperprolactinemia. Ther Clin Risk Manag. 2007;3(5):929–95.
18. Gupta AK, Madzia SE, Batra R. Etiology and management of Seborrheic dermatitis. Dermatology. 2004;208:89–93. https://doi.org/10.1159/000076478.
19. Kahana M, Grossman E, Feinstein A, Cohen M, Ronnen M, Millet MS. Skin tags: a cutaneous marker for diabetes mellitus. Acta Derma Venereol. 1987;67:175–7.
20. Tompkins RR. Skin tags and diabetes. Arch dermatol. 1977;133:1463.
21. Thappa DM. Skin tags as markers of diabetes mellitus: An epidemiological study in India. J Dermatol. 1995;22:729–31.
22. Bhargara P, Mathur D. Acrochordon, diabetes and associations. Indian J Dermal Veneriol Leprol. 1996;62:226–8.

23. Garcia-Hidalgo L, Orozco-Topete R, Gonzalez-BarrancoJ VAR, Dalman JJ, Ortiz-Pedroza G. Dermatoses in 156 obese adults. Obes Res. 1999;7:299–302.
24. Yamada GPEN, Bhawan L. Light microscopic immunohistochemical and ultrastructural alterations in patients with melasma. Am J Dermatopathol. 2005;27:96–101.
25. Perez M, Sanchez JL, Aguilo F. Endocrinology profile of patients with idiopathic melasma. Invest Dermatol. 1983;81:543.
26. Muzaffar F, Hassan I, et al. Physiologic skin changes during pregnancy. Int J Dermatol. 1998;37:429–31.
27. Anon. Res J Biol Sci. 2007;2(5):593–6.
28. Malek J, Chedraoui A, Nikolic D, Barouti N, Ghosn S, Abbas O. Successful treatment of hydroquinone-resistant melasma using topical methimazole. Dermatol Ther. 2013;26:69–72.
29. Zhong SM, Sun N, Liu HX, Niu YQ, Wu Y. Reduction of facial pigmentation of melasma by topical lignin peroxidase: a novel fast-acting skin-lightening agent. Exp Ther Med. 2015;9:341–4.
30. Lee JH, Park JG, Lim SH, Kim JY, Ahn KY, Kim MY, et al. Localized intradermal microinjection of tranexamic acid for treatment of melasma in Asian patients: a preliminary clinical trial. Dermatologic Surg. 2006;32:626–31.
31. Eimpunth E, Wanitphakdeedecha R, Triwongwaranat R, Varothai S, Manuskiatti W. Therapeutic outcome of melasma treatments by dual wavelength (511 and 578nm) laser in patients with skin phototypes 3 to 5. Clin Exp Dermatol. 2014;39:292–7.
32. Hilton S, Heise H, Buhren BA, Schrumpf H, Bolke E, et al. Treatment of melasma in Caucasion patients using a novel 694-nm Q switched ruby fractional laser. Eur J Med Res. 2013;18:43.
33. Radmanesh M, Azar-Beig M, et al. Burning, paradoxical hypertrichosis, leukotrichia and folliculitis are four major complications of intense pulsed light hair removal therapy. J Dermatolog Treat. 2008;19(6):360–3.

Chapter 10
Management of Hirsutism in PCOS

Rashmi Shetty and Meera Govindaraju

10.1 Introduction

Hirsutism is defined as excessive growth of terminal hair in androgen-dependent areas in women. It is one of the most used clinical criteria for the diagnosis of androgen levels, being observed in 50–80% of the patients with hyperandrogenism [1–3] (Fig. 10.1). However a small percentage of women can present with what is called as Idiopathic hirsutism with hyperandrogenism no detectable hormonal abnormality, normal ovaries and normal menstrual cycles.

Ferriman and Gallwey in 1961 used a method to clinically assess the degree and extent of hirsutism. Original scale assessed 11 different body zones—upper lip, chin, chest, upper and lower back, upper and lower abdomen, arm, forearms, thighs and lower legs with scores ranging from (0) with no visible terminal hair growth to (4) showing extensive visible hair growth for each body part being evaluated. A score ≥ 8 typically indicates hirsutism. The modified version scored nine body zones [excluding forearm and legs] and is the current gold standard [1, 4]. However the limiting factor is that it is subjective and shows inter-observer variation.

Patients without evident hirsutism can present with biochemical signs and ultrasound suggestive of severe PCOS in contrast there is another set of patients with severe hirsutism showing minor changes in biochemical values [5] This explains the variability in the inherent sensitivity of the pilosebaceous unit to androgens. Hence there is no correlation of the score with androgen levels [6–8].

R. Shetty (✉)
RA Clinics, Mumbai/Hyderabad, India
e-mail: Rashmi@drrashmishetty.com

M. Govindaraju
Chennai, India

R. Singh, N. Sharma (eds.), *A Guide to Hormonal Dermatology*,
https://doi.org/10.1007/978-981-99-7715-4_10

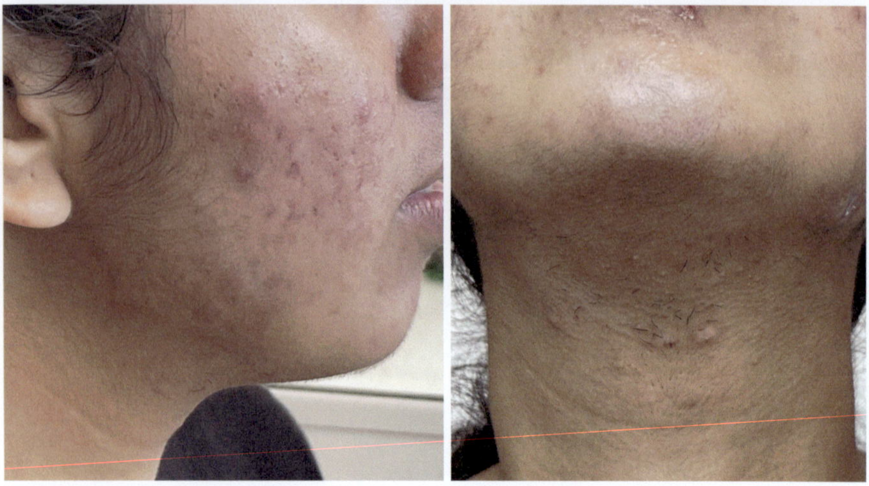

Fig. 10.1 Presence of terminal hairs in male pattern distribution with acne and seborrhea

Hair follicle sensitivity is determined by racial, ethnic, and genetic differences [9–11]. Hence influence hirsutism clinically. It's important to differentiate hirsutism from hypertrichosis as in the latter excess hair[vellus] growth occurs in non-androgenic areas. The occurrence of metabolic disorders and cardiovascular risk markers in women with hirsutism correlates with the severity of hyperandrogenemia.

10.1.1 Causes

Hirsutism can be

1. Idiopathic [normal androgen/normal ovarian function]
2. Androgen excess [tumours [ovarian/adrenal], PCOS]
3. Non classic adrenal hyperplasia
4. Increased sensitivity of hair follicles to androgens
5. Non androgenic factors—hereditary, medications (ref Table 10.1), metabolic disorders, chronic skin irritation [6]

As PCOS is primarily a diagnosis of exclusion its of prime importance to rule out other conditions that might mimic PCOS. Hence apart from measuring circulating androgens such as serum testosterone which may be normal to increased, other lab values like LH/FSH [13] ratio, Dehydroepiandrosterone sulfate (DHEAS)—Raised DHEAS (>700 μg/dL) indicates an adrenal cause, benign or malignant are checked. In cases of CAH—17 Hydroxy progesterone is measured. The measurement should be done between 0700 and 0900 h in the early follicular phase of the menstrual cycle. Levels less than 2 ng/mL excludes the disease. Mildly increased levels between 300 and 1000 ng/dL require an ACTH stimulation test. Cosyntropin [14]

Table 10.1 Common medications associated with Hirsutism and/or Hypertrichosis [12]

Hirsutism:
• Aripiprazole
• OCPs
• Bimatoprost
• Bupropion
• Carbamazepine
• Clonazepam
• Corticosteroids
• Cyclosporine
• Dantrolene
• Fluoxetine
• Interferon alfa
• Isotretinoin
• Diazoxide,
• Donepezil
• Eszopiclone
• Estrogens
• Fluoxetine
• interferon alpha
• Isotretinoin
• Lamotrigine
• Leuprolide
• Mycophenolate mofetil
• Olanzapine
• Paroxetine
• Pregabalin
• Progestins
• Selegiline
• Tacrolimus
• Testosterones
• Tiagabine
• Trazadone
• Venlafaxine
• Zonisamide
Hypertrichosis:
• Acitretin
• Azelaic acid
• Cetirizine
• Citalopram
• Corticosteroids
• Cyclosporine
• Etonogestrel implant
• Phenytoin

(synthetic ACTH), 250 μg, is administered intravenously, and levels of 17-hydroxy-progesterone are measured before and one hour after the injection. Post-stimulation values (>10 ng/mL) constitute a positive test. 24-h urine free cortisol to be checked in women with signs and symptoms of Cushing's syndrome. Increased prolactin levels seen in hyperprolactinemia due to hypothalamic disease or a pituitary tumour. A raised TSH level is seen in hypophyseal hypothyroidism [15] and it can act as a cofactor in hirsutism. So, its important to measure serum TSH levels.

10.1.2 Evaluation

History of onset—childhood/peripubertal, family history and racial history, history of drug intake (Table 10.1), menstrual history—dating back to puberty, hypertension, diabetes mellitus [Cushing's syndrome] and rapid weight gain to be considered.

10.1.3 Examination

Clinical assessment is done with modified Ferriman and Gallwey [4] scoring system. When we plan a treatment for hirsutism, it is important to examine the skin for active acne, condition of skin barrier, skin dryness, hypersensitivity, any local redness/inflammation and infection so as to make sure that we plan safer and better treatment protocol for the patient.

Points to note are severity of hirsutism correlates poorly with severity of androgen excess. The reason behind this paradox is that hirsutism not only reflects circulating androgens but is also influenced by peripheral metabolism of androgens and by insulin resistance and compensatory hyperinsulinemia.

There are certain limitations of current androgen assays (Table 10.2). So it's important to

1. Obtain at least one determination of serum androgen levels in patients with hirsutism before starting on treatment.

Table 10.2 Investigations for Hirsutism: (Hormonal profile)[16, 17]

Free testosterone	Most sensitive—ovarian origin
Total testosterone	
LH/FSH	>2.5 PCOS [18]—less sensitive
SHBG	
Fasting insulin levels	
DHEAs	To rule out CAH
Prolactin	Irregular menses/galactorrhea ↑
Serum progesterone	After DMST
Cortisol	After DMST
17OHP basal	>2 ng/mL early morning sample
17OHP ACTH	>10 ng/mL
ACTH	Late onset adrenal hyperplasia
Androstenedione	Ovarian cause
USG pelvis	Cystic ovaries
Lipid profile and TSH	
BMI/Waist circumference/BP	

Plasma hormone concentrations are determined during fasting in a specimen obtained during the first 7 days of the menstrual cycle: total and free testosterone, DHEAS, prolactin, LH and FSH, and 17-hydroxyprogesterone (17-OHP) Clinical BP is determined

2. Free testosterone remains the most sensitive [16] tool among the circulating androgens.
3. High quality direct double antibody radioimmunoassay for total testosterone or using LC/MS [16] techniques.
4. The diagnostic performance of measuring serum total testosterone is enhanced by the concomitant measurement of SHBG. Serum testosterone and SHBG levels have a high predictive [17] value for PCOS in epidemiologic studies. Also, serum SHBG is a useful surrogate marker [19] for insulin resistance.

10.2 Treatments

10.2.1 General Care

It is best to address the skin issues to get the skin to healthier situation, to repair the skin barrier, reduce the inflammation and make sure hydration of the skin is at its best and then plan for the laser therapy.

10.2.2 Topical Treatment

Eflorinithine [20]13.9% cream which causes irreversible inhibition of L-Ornithine decarboxylase the enzyme which controls hair growth and proliferation thereby slowly reducing the hair regrowth and makes it less evident. Twice daily application for a period of 8–24 weeks is recommended. Usage of this cream with other permanent hair reduction methods have proven to improve the overall outcome. However, there are certain limitations in using this topical as its inconvenient to use the product for months together and can prove comedogenic for a PCOS patient where the skin is already seborrheic due to hyperandrogenemia. And patient compliance is a big question in the new age skin care routine.

10.2.3 Oral Treatment

Treatment of hyperandrogenism is directed at:

1. suppressing androgen production in the ovaries and adrenal glands
2. reducing the level of bioavailable androgens
3. inhibiting the conversion of weaker androgens to more potent forms; and
4. decreasing the activity of androgens on receptors in target tissues.

Table 10.3 OCP-Mechanism of action

EE-CPA	Suppresses ovarian androgen synthesis by inhibition of gonadotrophin secretion from the pituitary
EE-DROSP	
EE-Norgestimate	Estrogen increases the hepatic synthesis of SHBG, thus suppresses the free testosterone levels

Table 10.4 Progestins and anti-androgen potency [23]

Progestins with low androgenic activity	Progestins with high androgenic activity
Desogestrel	Cyproterone acetate
Gestodene	Chlormadinone acetate
Norgestimate	Drosperinone—SPA derivative
	Dienogest Nogestrel
	Levonorgestrel
	Normalizes testosterone levels

10.2.3.1 Myoinostiol

Both Myoinositol [21] and D-chiro-inositol (MDI) reduce insulin resistance, reduces androgen levels (testosterone and androstenedione), corrects the LH/FSH ratio there by improves ovarian function in PCOS. DMI also reduces lipids, and blood pressure. Chromium picolinate [22] (CrP) a mineral is also useful in reducing the insulin resistance (IR). These also help in reducing LH hormones.

10.2.3.2 Oral Contraceptive Pills

Estrogens with progestins is the mainstay of treatment and is especially recommended for women not interested in conception. Hence useful as an effective contraception and paves way for treating with concomitant antiandrogens for regularizing the cycles as well (Tables 10.3 and 10.4).

10.3 Anti Androgens

No FDA labeling for treatment of hirsutism.

10.3.1 Cyproterone Acetate [24]

CPA antagonizes the effect of androgens at the peripheral level. It decreases the circulating testosterone and androstenedione levels through a decrease in serum LH levels. Usually given on day 1 or day 5 for 10 days per month in a dose of 50–100 mg/day. Side effects include Adrenal insufficiency or loss of libido.

10.3.2 Spironolactone

Potassium sparing diuretic, works by competitive inhibition of the androgen receptors/5 alpha reductase activity. The combination of spironolactone with OCs [25] commonly used with effective results.

Dose: 25–100 mg twice a day for 6–12 months significantly reduced hirsutism. Blood pressure and potassium monitoring is essential during initial therapy. SPA needs to be taken along with food as this increases its absorption [26] and prevents gastritis.

10.3.3 Flutamide/Bicalutamide [27]

Nonsteroidal androgen receptor blocker.

Dosage: 250 mg–500 mg/day. Hepatoxicity and renal failure limits its usage.

10.3.4 Finasteride/Dutasteride

Competitive inhibitor of 5 alpha reductase type 2 enzyme.

Dose: 1–5 mg/day. However, all anti androgens are contraindicated during pregnancy as feminization of male fetus can occur. Hence are prescribed to women ready to use contraceptive methods.

Anti androgens are usually indicated for moderate to severe hirsutism or mild hirsutism not responding to treatment with OCPs even after a year (Table 10.5).

10.3.4.1 Glucocorticoids

GC Suppress adrenal androgens but its usage is of little concern in women with PCOS as it has its deleterious effect on lipid and glucose metabolism. Unless a significant adrenal androgen excess requires its usage.

10.3.4.2 GnRH Analogues

Leuprolide and Naferelin reduce LH and testosterone, increases FSH and SHBG thus improving the hirsutism. Reversible loss of bone mineral density is of concern. Ovarian hyperandrogenism refractory [29] to hormonal therapy calls for usage of GnRH analogues.

Table 10.5 Anti androgens (dosage) [28]

CPA–50–100 mg/day
Spironolactone –25–100 mg/day
Flutamide—250—500 mg/day
Finasteride—1–5 mg/day

10.3.4.3 Insulin Sensitizers

Metformin lowers the insulin levels and hence the circulating androgen levels. Decreases the androgen production by theca cells and has a direct effect on ovarian steroidogenesis but does not help with hirsutism compared to its usage in reducing the insulin resistance. Initial dose is 500 mg given during dinner time and can be increased every week until a maximum dose of 2000 mg/day divided in two doses can be given. They are beneficial in reducing the BMI and in regularizing the menstrual cycle. Side effects include GI discomfort.

Thiazolidinedione—Troglitazone, rosiglitazone, and pioglitazone all three work by reducing insulin levels and suppresses the androgen production in ovary and adrenals. Among this troglitazone showed significant result in hirsutism but was withdrawn due to hepatotoxicity.

10.3.4.4 Antifungal Agents

Ketoconazole [30] is an imidazole derivative that is used as a broad-spectrum antifungal agent that reduces androgen production in the testes and the adrenal glands. Oral ketoconazole in the dose of 400 mg daily has also been tried for few cases. However hepatic toxicity necessitates regular monitoring of liver function.

10.3.5 Alternative Therapies [31]

There are a whole group of plant derived anti androgens that might be useful to reduce the androgen levels in PCOS with fewer side effects. They are good complementary therapies that occur naturally. These are as follows:

- Red reishi also known as Lingzhi in Chinese a mushroom species which reduces the 5 alpha reductase levels hence preventing the conversion of testosterone.
- Licorice/Glycyrrhiza glabra -which contains phytoestrogens mimics the estrogens effect and reduces the testosterone levels.
- Green tea—epigallocatechins present in the green tea can inhibit the 5 alpha reductase and act as anti-androgens.
- Spearmint or Mentha spicata—a herbal remedy seems to reduce the free testosterone without affecting the total testosterone or DHEAS levels.
- Saw palmetto/Serenoa repens is a small palm tree extract and is an effective anti-androgen as it contains phytosterols.

Cosmetic treatment of hirsutism includes both temporary and permanent methods. Temporary methods include bleaching, waxing, plucking, shaving, plucking and depilatories. However, bleaching may leave a whole tuft of golden hair which might not be aesthetically pleasing, and frequent shaving can lead to razor bumps, folliculitis and sensitive skin as well.

10.4 In-Clinic Treatment

10.4.1 Electrolysis [32]

First described in the year 1875. It is a technique wherein a needle is accurately inserted into the hair follicle with certain intensity and duration thereby destroying hair follicle. Anagen hairs are targeted hence hairs are shaved 1–5 days prior to the procedure. Usually, a blend method which includes passing of direct current [galvanic electrolysis] and high frequency alternate current [destructive thermolysis] is used in this method. If competently performed it does not cause any scar. This method works best for few hairs or if hirsutism is manifested in a localized area. So, it is wise to choose this method of treatment than lasers as the latter can lead to paradoxical hair growth of the surrounding hair which maybe vellus and absorb inadequate energy. However transient side effects like discomfort, post inflammatory erythema, pigmentation, occasional wheals or small crusts can develop. Prior application of topical anesthetic reduces the discomfort to a great extent.

10.4.2 Lasers and Lights

Lasers or laser heat energy-based devices cause long term hair reduction. These lasers operate in the red or near-infrared wavelengths and rely on selective photothermolysis [33] the target being melanin pigment leading to hair follicle destruction.

Various lasers for hair removal include diode, ruby, alexandrite, Q-switched yttrium-aluminium-garnet [YAG] and intense pulsed light therapy.

10.4.3 Mechanisms of Lasers

Selective thermolysis enables us to target the melanin chromophore present in the hair shaft. However, for a heterogenous structure like a pigmented hair follicle it requires diffusion of heat from chromophore to the desired target for complete destruction. This is called extended [34]theory of selective photothermolysis.

Certain key variables like wavelength, spot size, pulse width and skin cooling, compression are important determinants for the best outcome of any laser for hair reduction without undue side effects.

- Longer wavelengths have better penetration.
- Higher fluences for thicker hair or lower fluence with multiple passes[SHR] gives optimal results.
- Spot size wider than 6 mm helps in faster coverage of larger areas. One can either modify the energy and the spot size if you have one kind of laser or along the

cycle of the hair, there is transfer, terminal to vellus hair different kinds of lasers can be used for the same patient for optimum results.

- Longer pulse durations are preferred as there is faster dissipation of heat from the epidermis. Perifollicular edema and erythema [35] are the desired clinical end points. Patients with light skin and dark hair respond well to LHR. Diode lasers [36] 800–810 nm are more reliable than other lasers. They come with sapphire tip with cooling capacity. Long pulsed [36] neodymium:yag laser [1064 nm] is recommended for type 4,5 and 6 skin types. Their longer wavelength gives better penetration.
- Diode and alexandrite lasers appear to be more effective than intense pulsed light,neodymium:YAG or ruby lasers. Type 2 skin responds better to alexandrite and diode lasers. Long pulsed alexandrite 755 nm [37] works well on type 1 to 4 skin types. Ruby [694 nm] has been reported to show more post inflammatory hyperpigmentation in dark skin.
- Treatment with IPL is useful for lighter hairs, but more sessions are required and recurrence is not uncommon within an year. Any age above 16 years. lasers for hair reduction can be started in other words when secondary sexual characteristics develop and there is presence of excessive terminal hair warrants treatment with lasers.

10.5 Conclusion

Hirsutism could be in one part or in multiple parts of the body so lasers with large spot size as in new age laser could be used as larger body surface could be covered in short duration whereas lasers with smaller spot size which is time consuming for a patient, areas like face, neck, arm, and legs can be tackled first and rest of the body areas can follow. Also, its important to set the expectations right in saying as the number of sessions may not be necessarily between 8 to 10 and might need much more sessions depending upon the outcome of the hair growth as monitored with regular visits. Patients weight loss and PCOS journey along with strict adherence to oral medications needs to be monitored. It's essential to emphasize to the patient that treating the basic cause is important. Monitoring the PCOS in terms of lab work and lifestyle modification with weight loss may really add value to those disgruntled patients who might come back after 10–12 sessions with no reduction in hair growth. Monitoring the energy and shift of the core laser might be important as treatment progresses from a terminal to less hairs. In most aesthetic clinic, lasers are done by trained technicians under the supervision of doctors but however along the way if the hair density, thickness or the color of the hair, terminal or vellus hair is looked up and the energy or the laser has to be changed accordingly to benefit the patient. Counselling the patient about the skin care and other topical cream usage in between laser sessions also helps in getting the best possible aesthetic outcome for the patient. An evidence-based strategies and treatment of the underlying cause together benefits the patients in the long run.

References

1. Hatch R, Rosenfield RL, Kim MH, Tredway D. Hirsutism: implications, etiology, and management. Am J Obstet Gynecol. 1981;140:815–30.
2. Lee AT, Zane LT. Dermatologic manifestations of polycystic ovary syndrome. Am J Clin Dermatol. 2007;8:201–19.
3. Yildiz BO. Diagnosis of hyperandrogenism: clinical criteria. Best Pract Res Clin Endocrinol Metab. 2006;20:167–76.
4. Ferriman D, Gallwey JD. Clinical assessment of body hair growth in women. J Clin Endocrinol Metab. 1961;21:1440–7.
5. Goldzieher JW, Young RL. Selected aspects of polycystic ovarian disease. Endocrinol Metab Clin N Am. 1992;21:141–71.
6. Martin KA, Chang RJ, Ehrmann DA, Ibanez L, Lobo RA, Rosenfield RL, et al. Evaluation and treatment of hirsutism in premenopausal women: an endocrine society clinical practice guideline. J Clin Endocrinol Metab. 2008;93:1105–20.
7. Lobo RA, Goebelsmann U, Horton R. Evidence for the importance of peripheral tissue events in the development of hirsutism in polycystic ovary syndrome. J Clin Endocrinol Metab. 1983;57:393–7.
8. Reingold SB, Rosenfield RL. The relationship of mild hirsutism or acne in women to androgens. Arch Dermatol. 1987;123:209–12.
9. Deplewski D, Rosenfield RL. Role of hormones in pilosebaceous unit develop–45. Endocr Rev. 2000;21(4):363–92.
10. Carmina E, Koyama T, Chang L, et al. Does ethnicity influence the prevalence of adrenal hyperandrogenism and insulin resistance in polycystic ovary syndrome. Am J Obstet Gynecol. 1992;167(6):1807–12.
11. Ehrmann DA, Rosenfield RL. Clinical review 10: an endocrinologic approach to the patient with hirsutism. J Clin Endocrinol Metab. 1990;71(1):1–4.
12. Physicians' Desk Reference Web site. http://www.pdr.net. Accessed 13 Apr 2011.
13. Chang RJ, Katz SE. Diagnosis of polycystic ovary syndrome. Endocrinol Metab Clin N Am. 1999;28:397–408.
14. New MI, Lorenzen F, Lerner AJ, et al. Genotyping steroid 21-hydroxylase deficiency: hormonal reference data. J Clin Endocrinol Metab. 1983;57:320–6.
15. Schmidt JB, Lindmaier A, Spona J. Hyperprolactinemia and hypophyseal hypothyroidism as cofactors in hirsutism and androgen-induced alopecia in women. Hautarzt. 1991;42:168–72.
16. Azziz R, Carmina E, Dewailly D, Diamanti-Kandarakis E, Escobar-Morreale HF, Futterweit W, Janssen OE, Legro RS, Norman RJ, Taylor AE, et al. The androgen excess and PCOS Society criteria for the polycystic ovary syndrome: the complete task force report. Fertil Steril. 2009;91:456–88.
17. Escobar-Morreale HF, Asuncion M, Calvo RM, Sancho J, San Millan JL. Receiver operating characteristic analysis of the performance of basal serum hormone profiles for the diagnosis of polycystic ovary syndrome in epidemiological studies. Eur J Endocrinol. 2001;145:619–24.
18. Steinberger E, Smith KD, Rodriguez-Rigau LJ. Hyperandrogenism and female infertility. In: Crogsignani PG, Rubin B, editors. Endocrinology of human infertility: new aspects. London: Academic Press; 1981. p. 327–42.
19. Pugeat M, Crave JC, Tourniaire J, Forest MG. Clinical utility of sex hormone-binding globulin measurement. Horm Res. 1996;45:148–55.
20. Barman Balfour JA, McClellan K. Topical Eflornithine. Am J Clin Dermatol. 2001;2:197–201.
21. Papaleo E, Unfer V, Baillargeon JP, De Santis L, Fusi F, Brigante C. Myo-inositol in patients with polycystic ovary syndrome : a novel method for ovulation induction. Gynecol Endocrinol. 2007;23:700–3.
22. Anon. J Obstet Gynaecol Res. 2016;42(3):279–85. https://doi.org/10.1111/jog.12907. Epub 2015 Dec 14.

23. Porcile A, Gallardo E. Long-term treatment of hirsutism: desogestrel compared with cyproterone acetate in oral contraceptives. Fertil Steril. 1991;55:877–81.
24. van der Spuy ZM, le Roux PA. Cyproterone acetate for hirsutism. Cochrane Database Syst Rev. 2003;10:CD001125.
25. Pittaway DE, Maxson WS, Wentz AC. Spironolactone in combination drug therapy for unresponsive hirsutism. Fertil Steril. 1985;43:878–82.
26. Spritzer PM, Lisboa KO, Mattiello S, Lhullier F. Spironolactone as a single agent for long-term therapy of hirsute patients. Clin Endocrinol. 2000;52:587–94.
27. Castelo-Branco C, Del Pino M. Hepatotoxicity during low-dose flutamide treatment for hirsutism. Gynecol Endocrinol. 2009;25:419–22.
28. Moghetti P, Tosi F, Tosti A, Negri C, Misciali C, Perrone F, Caputo M, Muggeo M, Castello R. Comparison of spironolactone, flutamide, and finasteride efficacy in the treatment of hirsutism: a randomized, double blind, placebo-controlled trial. J Clin Endocrinol Metab. 2000a;85:89–94.
29. de Leo V, Fulghesu AM, la Marca A, Morgante G, Pasqui L, Talluri B, et al. Hormonal and clinical effects of GnRH agonist alone, or in combination with a combined oral contraceptive or flutamide in women with severe hirsutism. Gynecol Endocrinol. 2000;14:411–6.
30. Venturoli S, Marescalchi O, Colombo FM, Macrelli S, Ravaioli B, Bagnoli A, Paradisi R, Flamigni C. A prospective randomized trial comparing low dose flutamide, finasteride, ketoconazole, and cyproterone acetate-estrogen regimens in the treatment of hirsutism. J Clin Endocrinol Metab. 1999;84:1304–10.
31. Anon. Int J Endocrinol Metab. 2012;10(2):497–502. https://doi.org/10.5812/ijem.3644.
32. Anon. J Am Acad Dermatol. 1995;33(4):662–6. https://doi.org/10.1016/0190-9622(95)91290-8.
33. Anderson RR, Parrish JA. Selective photothermolysis: precise microsurgery by selective absorption of pulsed radiation. Science. 1983;220:524–52.
34. Altshuler G, Anderson R, Manstein D, et al. Extended theory of selective photothermolysis. Laser Surg Med. 2001;29(5):416–32.
35. Ibrahimi O, Avram M, Hanke C, et al. Laser hair removal. Dermatol Ther. 2011;24(1):94–107.
36. Buddhadev R, Kirane V. Laser and light–assisted hair removal. In: Venkataram M, editor. ACSI Textbook on Cutaneous and Aesthetic surgery. 1st ed. Delhi: JP Brothers Medical Publishers Pvt. Ltd; 2012. p. 771–86.
37. Eremia S, Li C, Newman N. Laser hair removal with alexandrite versus diode laser using four treatment sessions. Dermatologic Surg. 2001;27(11):925–30.

Chapter 11
PCOS-Management of Androgenetic Alopecia

A. S. Savitha and R. Raghunatha Reddy

11.1 Introduction

Polycystic ovary syndrome (PCOS) is the most common endocrine disorder affecting women of reproductive age, involving pathways that produce metabolic, reproductive, cardiovascular and dermatologic effects. Around 4–20% of Indian women in the reproductive age group may have problems related to PCOS, in fact the actual problem is much more than what has been reported as per the experience of the clinicians [1]. The complaints that women with PCOS commonly face are irregularities in menstrual periods, oligomenorrhoea, hirsutism, and acne and hair loss. Many women with PCOS have polycystic appearance of ovaries on ultrasonography examination. Hair loss in women can be either telogen effluvium which is diffuse or female pattern hair loss (FPHL), where the loss is seen more on the frontal area. FPHL is specifically reported as a clinical sign of hyperandrogenism associated with PCOS. FPHL is progressive nonscarring type of alopecia. Although the exact incidence of alopecia in PCOS is not clear, approximately 20–30% of women with PCOS have troublesome hair loss [2]. It is generally associated with other symptoms like hirsutism, acanthosis nigricans or acne. Hair loss as a sole complaint is rare in PCOS. Recent guidelines on the diagnosis of polycystic ovary syndrome (PCOS) continue using the more general term "alopecia" and consider the finding diagnostic for the presence of hyperandrogenism [3]. The relationship of hair loss and androgen excess in women is neither consistent nor clear.

A. S. Savitha
Roots Institute of Dermatologic Sciences, Bangalore, India

Department of Dermatology, Sapthagiri Institute of Medical Sciences, Bangalore, India

R. R. Reddy (✉)
Department of Dermatology, Sapthagiri Institute of Medical Sciences, Bangalore, India

R. Singh, N. Sharma (eds.), *A Guide to Hormonal Dermatology*,
https://doi.org/10.1007/978-981-99-7715-4_11

The two most common types of female pattern hair loss seen in PCOS are

(a) Ludwig pattern: When there is thinning of hair over the central part of the top of the head (vertex) with preservation of frontal hair line
(b) Olsen pattern: There is accentuated loss of hair in the frontal part around the central hair parting line, which gives a Christmas tree pattern of hair loss

Male pattern hair loss, with the receding of the frontal hair line and temporal (on sides) balding, is rare in PCOS and should incite a search for other causes of hormonal imbalance.

11.1.1 Pathogenesis

The pilosebaceous unit is responsive to different hormones, especially the male hormones (like testosterone). In PCOS, there is hyperandrogenemia. This disturbance is accentuated by weight gain. The mechanism by which androgens cause hair loss has been linked to increased production of cytokines, which induce the hair to enter the telogen phase and the dermal papilla to become senescent. Under the influence of male hormones, the pilo-sebaceous unit shrinks (miniaturization) which leads to thinning and early fall of hair. The androgen receptor (AR) and three important enzymes, 5alpha-reductase I, II, and aromatase, are present in the outer root sheath and dermal papillae of hair follicles. The AR content in female frontal hair follicles is 40% lower than that in the male follicles. Frontal hair follicles in women have 3 and 3.5 times less 5alpha-reductase I and II levels, respectively. However, aromatase content in frontal hair is six times higher in women. This may, in part, explain the difference in clinical expression of hair loss between men and women.

11.2 Investigations

For PCOS, biochemical investigations may be normal. Nevertheless, women with signs of hirsutism, moderate to severe and/or treatment-refractory adult acne, acanthosis nigricans, irregular menses, oligomenorrhoea, and or galactorrhea should be screened for androgen excess.

Free and/or total Testosterone and DHEA-S are indispensable biochemical parameters Serum prolactin levels may also be elevated. If Testosterone is greater than 2.5 times of normal or > 200 ng/dL, or DHEA-S is greater than 2 times or > 700 g/dL in pre-menopausal or > 400 g/dL in post-menopausal women, imaging should be undertaken for possible underlying neoplasm.

Investigations for other causes for hair loss also should be undertaken like thyroid tests, Vit D and Vit B12 levels, iron deficiency.

11.3 Management

Management of hair fall in PCOS involves the following strategies:

- Non-pharmacologic: Maintaining a healthy weight with proper diet and exercise helps to mitigate all symptoms of PCOS.
- Pharmacologic:
  - *Oral contraceptive pills*: These are the mainstay of the management of PCOS. These hormonal pills help to reduce the androgen (male hormones) production from the ovaries and help in reducing hair fall. Most side effects are mild and disappear after continued use or change to other preparation. These minor side effects include bleeding in between the periods, nausea, vomiting, abdominal cramps, breast tenderness etc.
  - *Anti-Androgen Therapy*: Due to their propensity to cause feminization of the male fetus, They are contra-indicated in pregnant women and it is advisable to combine them with oral contraceptive pills (OCPs), especially in pre-menopausal women.

11.3.1 5 Alpha-Reductase Inhibitors

Although compared with men, women have lower levels of this enzyme in the dermal papilla; inhibitors of this enzyme have been found to be effective in arresting hair loss in FPHL.

11.3.1.1 Finasteride

Finasteride, an inhibitor of 5alpha-reductase type II enzyme, suppresses systemic as well as hair follicular androgen activity by inhibiting conversion of testosterone to its more active form, that is, dihydroxy testosterone (DHT). Finasteride is often used in women with FPHL, especially when hyperandrogenism is present. The efficacy of this drug in FPHL has been reported to be variable in different studies. Finasteride is generally well-tolerated. Infrequent side-effects in female patients include breast tenderness, which are most common in the first year of therapy and tend to diminish with continued use. Whenever used in pre-menopausal women, it should always be combined with OCPs or other effective method of contraception to prevent inadvertent conception and feminization of male fetus.

Dose of 2.5 mg to 5 mg is recommended for duration of at least one year and may be continued for few more months if deemed necessary.

11.3.1.2 Dutasteride

Dutasteride, an inhibitor of both type I and type II 5 alpha reductase, has been found to be more effective than finasteride in men with MPHL. Dutasteride has a much longer half-life than finasteride, and women of child-bearing potential should avoid its use without effective contraception for at least 6 months after discontinuation owing to its potential teratogenic effect. Dutasteride inhibits both type I and type II 5alpha -reductase enzyme and is three times more potent blocker of type II enzyme.

(a) ***Spironolactone:*** Spironolactone, an anti-androgen, is often used for treating hirsutism, acne, and seborrhea It is a potassium-sparing diuretic. Spironolactone works by blocking the action of the male hormones on their receptors on the pilosebaceous unit. It also has some effect in reducing the synthesis of androgens. It is mostly used in combination with OC pills, and doses of 100 to 200 mg/d and prolonged treatments (at least 12 months) are needed. Hair regrowth or stabilization of hair loss is observed in a variable number of patients. It is relatively safe, however some patients may have postural dizziness, especially on getting up quickly from lying down position. Few patients may have inter menstrual spotting as a common side effect. It may increase the frequency of micturition and rarely can increase the blood potassium levels. In a study where eighty women with biopsy-proven FPHL were studied, most without biochemical hyperandrogenism; 40 received spironolactone 200 mg daily, and 40 received cyproterone acetate. Both drugs were found to be effective. A combination of spironolactone and 5% minoxidil has also been found to be efficacious.

(b) **Flutamide:** This is one of the most powerful anti-androgens having beneficial effect in treating alopecia. It works by inhibiting the uptake of androgen in the cells and blocking their receptors thereby reducing their effect. It is also reported to reduce androgen levels. Some patients (3 in 10,000) may develop potentially life threatening complication of liver failure. Hence it is no longer used for the treatment of alopecia in PCOS anymore.

11.3.2 Cyproterone Acetate

Cyproterone acetate is an antiandrogen used at high doses (50–100 mg/d) for hyperandrogenic women with FPHL with mixed results. This drug blocks ARs and inhibits gonadotropin- releasing hormone. It is available in combination with estradiol as an OCP. The beneficial role of cyproterone acetate (CPA) in isolation or in combination with OCPs in reducing hair shedding and increasing hair density is known and seems to be greater in patients with evidence of hyperandrogenism. In two studies using *Diane-35* for 6–9 months and as 2 mg CPA plus 50 mg ethinylestradiol daily plus additional 20 mg CPA on days 5–20 of the menstrual cycle, respectively, decrease in shedding and thinning of hair were observed [4]. In yet another study, pre-menopausal women received CPA 100 mg daily for the first 10 days of each menstrual cycle for 12 months in combination with an oral contraceptive, while post-menopausal women received 50 mg daily of CPA continuously. At the end of 12 months, 35 (44%) women had clearly visible hair regrowth, 35 (44%) had no change in hair density, and 10 (12%) had reduced hair density [5].

The overall balance of evidence supports a role for CPA in FPHL, especially in presence of hyperandrogenism. The most effective treatment dose seems to be 100 mg/day on days 5–15 of the menstrual cycle supplemented by 50 mg ethinylestradiol on days 5–25 [6].The adverse effects include menstrual disturbances, weight gain, loss of libido, depression, Breast tenderness and gastrointestinal upsets.

Drospirenone: A 17alpha-spironolactone derivative possesses progestagenic, anti-androgenetic, and antialdosteronic activities. It is administered in a dose of 3 mg/day in combination with 30 mg of ethinylestradiol during a 21-day cycle. It has been recommended for the treatment of SAHA and is devoid of fluid retention property.

11.4 Minoxidil

Oral minoxidil is being used increasingly in androgenetic alopecia. The dose ranges from 0.25 to 5 mg daily to twice daily. Successful treatment of female pattern hair loss, chronic telogen effluvium, monilethrix, and permanent chemotherapy-induced alopecia was also reported. The most common adverse effects with oral minoxidil included hypertrichosis and postural hypotension.

A common precaution to be followed while using any of the anti-androgen medications is to avoid getting pregnant while using them as they can cause abnormalities in genital development of male fetuses. However, these medications are generally used in combination with OC pills.

11.5 Topical Therapy

11.5.1 Minoxidil

Minoxidil is the only FDA approved topical therapy for hair loss. Minoxidil is the primary treatment for hair loss due to its mitogenic effects on hair follicles. It is a potassium channel opener and it enhances angiogenesis around the follicle, thereby increasing the blood supply to follicle. Minoxidil shortens the telogen phase, resulting in premature entry of resting hair follicles into the anagen phase. The anagen phase is also prolonged and miniaturized follicles are enlarged with minoxidil, resulting in increased hair counts, weight, and density.

It thus increases the hair count and volume. Minoxidil is available in lotion and foam preparation, 2% and 5% strengths. In women, only 2% minoxidil solutions are FDA approved. It is preferable to use 1 ml of 5% minoxidil twice daily only dry scalp for a minimum of 12 months. During the initial treatment period of 2–8 weeks, there can be a transient increase in scalp hair shedding, which results from the shedding of telogen hairs in preparation for new anagen growth. Treatment side effects are uncommon and include allergic or irritative contact dermatitis, which is more commonly related to the solution vehicle propylene glycol. This can be overcome by using the foam preparation. Another possible side effect is hypertrichosis of the forehead or face, usually caused by improper application.

Combinations with minoxidil are also being used increasingly.

A study showed that minoxidil and spironolactone, an aldosterone receptor blocker, in combination are an effective treatment option for FPHL [7]. Topical finasteride, which prevents the conversion of testosterone to dihydrotestosterone, and minoxidil combination therapy are also effective in treating FPHL. Other studies have shown that sublingual minoxidil is an effective method in treating hair loss due to the circumvention of hepatic metabolism by this route. This method increases the drugs' bioavailability when compared to its oral counterpart [8].

11.6 Lasers and Light Treatments

Low-level laser therapy is a relatively new treatment option that is an alternative to medical and surgical treatments. Lasers and light treatments are monochromatic lights that utilize wavelengths between 600–1400 nm, in the red/infrared spectrum. The light treatments can stimulate hair growth and can be used to manage FPHL. Laser therapy has minimal risks; studies have shown that it induces hair growth and thickness. Red or near-infrared laser light has been reported to promote tissue repair and regeneration and, more recently, low-intensity light laser (LLL) therapy has been demonstrated to stimulate hair growth, probably by increasing the mitotic rate of the hair follicle stem cells or follicular keratinocytes. Additionally, LLL may modulate inflammation by increasing TGF-b1 and IL-10 while reducing proinflammatory cytokines and prostaglandin E2. Several studies have shown that LLL may improve FPHL but the effect is generally modest and, in a male study, although hair count increased, no differences with global photographs were observed. Adverse effects are few but may include headache, erythema, pruritus, burning, pain, and mild paresthesia.

11.7 Invasive Procedures

11.7.1 Platelet Rich Plasma Therapy

Platelet rich plasma (PRP) is used effectively in the management of FPHL. Each session is repeated 4 weeks apart for 4–6 times. Platelet-rich plasma (PRP) is produced by centrifuging a patient's own blood, concentrating the platelets to ≥10,00,000/L, and injecting the concentrate into the patient's scalp in affected areas. In addition to platelets, PRP contains numerous growth factors, chemokines, and cytokines (Figs 11.1 and 11.2).

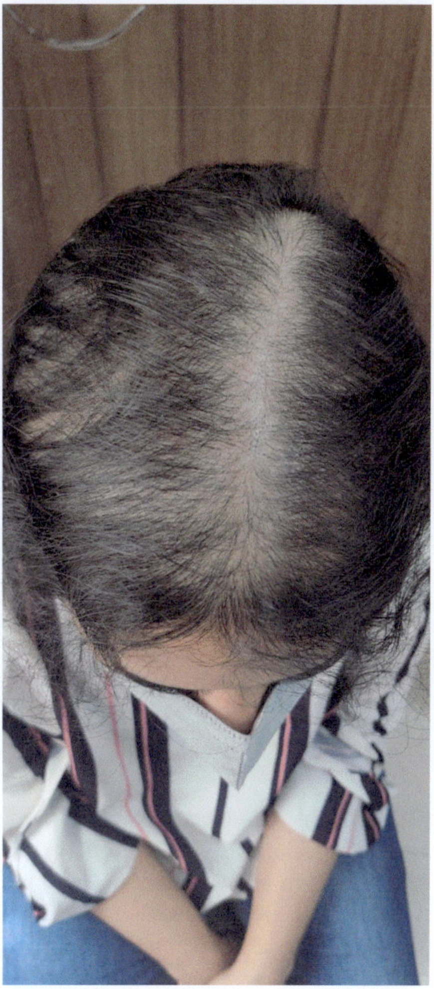

Fig. 11.1 PCOS with female pattern hair loss, frontal thinning with hairline maintained.

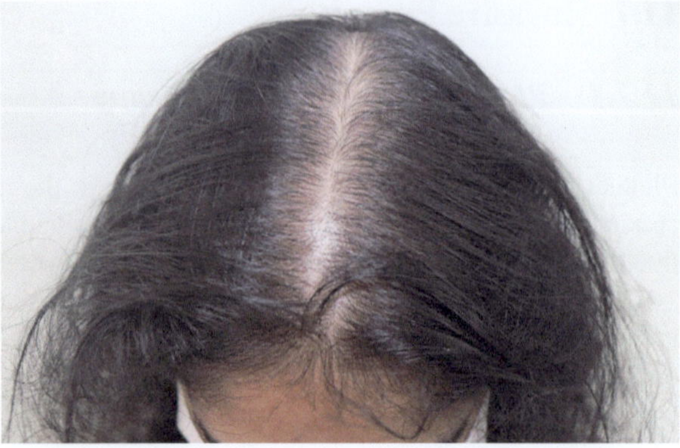

Fig. 11.2 Response seen after oral antiandrogens and 4 sittings of platelet rich plasma therapy

11.8 Microneedling

Tiny needles are rolled over areas of hair loss to puncture the skin. Using this technique with other treatments, such as minoxidil or platelet rich plasma, can allow the medication to penetrate deeper into the skin. The technique causes microtrauma that induces neovascularization, collagen formation, and stimulation of growth factors to increase hair growth and thickness.

11.9 Hair Transplantation

Hair transplantation is a beneficial method for cases of FPHL in individuals over the age of 25 who are unresponsive to alternative treatments, such as topical therapy or platelet rich plasma. The underling hormonal imbalance should be rectified before undertaking this procedure. In women with FPHL, hair transplantation may also be useful although the hair loss process, as in men, will continue outside of the transplant areas, so continued use of medical treatment after surgery is necessary.

11.10 Cosmetic Camouflage

Camouflaging products and other concealment techniques can effectively mask areas of visible hair loss. Hair fibers (keratin-made), masking lotions, topical shading, and scalp spray thickeners may be used. These are compatible with topical minoxidil and are easily removed with shampooing. Integration hairpiece (fabric- or skin-like material) or wig may used.

11.11 Conclusion

PCOS is a state of hyperandrogenemia, resulting in patterned hair loss in women. The management should include treatment of underlying disorder and specific treatment for hair loss.

References

1. Malik S, Jain K, Talwar P, Prasad S, Dhorepatil B, Devi G, Khurana A, et al. Management of polycystic ovary syndrome in India. Fertil Sci Res. 2014;1:23–43.
2. Carmina E, Azziz R, Bergfeld W, Escobar-Morreale HF, Futterweit W, et al. Female pattern hair loss and androgen excess: a report from the multidisciplinary androgen excess and PCOS committee. J Clin Endocrinol Metabol. 2019;104(7):2875–91. https://doi.org/10.1210/jc.2018-02548.
3. Odhaib SA, Al Hamdi K, Mansour AA. Is there any association between clinical and biochemical hyperandrogenism in women with female pattern hair loss? Cureus. 2020;12(11):1.
4. Brzezińska-Wcisło L. Assessment of efficacy of Diane-35 in androgenetic feminine alopecia. Wiadomosci Lekarskie. 2003;56(3–4):202–5.
5. Vexiau P, Chaspoux C, Boudou P, Fiet J, Jouanique C, Hardy N, Reygagne P. Effects of minoxidil 2% vs. cyproterone acetate treatment on female androgenetic alopecia: a controlled, 12-month randomized trial. Br J Dermatol. 2002;146(6):992–9.
6. Dawber RP, Sonnex T, Ralfs I. Oral antiandrogen treatment of common baldness in women. Br J Dermatol. 1982;107(suppl 22):20.
7. Burns LJ, De Souza B, Flynn E, et al. spironolactone for treatment of female pattern hair loss. J Am Acad Dermatol. 2020;s0190-9622:30510–7.
8. Sinclair R, de Carvalho l, Ismail F, et al. Treatment of male and female pattern hair loss with sublingual minoxidil: a retrospective case-series of 64 patients. J Eur Acad Dermatol Venereol. 2020;34:795. https://doi.org/10.1111/jdv.16616.

Chapter 12
Counselling in Hair Transplant Patient

Viral Desai

12.1 Introduction

Hair restoration is considered one of the most exciting and innovative surgical fields in cosmetic surgery today and with modern methods of graft harvesting and implantation, hair transplantation results represent a harmonious blend of art and science.

Hair transplantation is a surgical procedure which involves relocation or transfer of hairs from the occipital area of the scalp to the bald or thinning areas.

Follicular unit hair transplantation is a type of surgical hair restoration in which follicular units of hair, (consisting of naturally occurring bundles of hairs), are dissected under a stereomicroscope and transplanted in the bald area to give natural look.

Mini-micro-grafting is another method of hair transplantation involving randomly assorted groups of hairs, without consideration of their natural configuration of follicular units, under loupe or naked eye examination. Mini-grafts consist of 4-5-6 hairs while micro-grafts consist of 1–3 hairs [1].

Punch transplantation is a method of hair transplantation using punch grafts extracted from occipital area and transplanted into recipient sites created by punches. This method gives fairly cosmetically unacceptable results and is rarely used now [2].

Hair transplant consultations are essential preoperative assessments where the surgeon evaluates the patient's suitability for the procedure, discusses the available options, and provides advice on postoperative care. This article will give an overview of hair transplant basics and consultation.

V. Desai (✉)
CPLSS, Sarla Hospital/Desai Hospitals Pvt Ltd, Mumbai, Maharashtra, India
e-mail: drviral@drviraldesai.com

R. Singh, N. Sharma (eds.), *A Guide to Hormonal Dermatology*,
https://doi.org/10.1007/978-981-99-7715-4_12

The history of hair transplant dates back to the 1930s when Japanese surgeons first attempted to transplant hair in humans. However, the modern hair transplant technique was developed in the 1950s by Dr. Norman Orentreich [3]. Since then, hair transplant surgery has evolved, and new techniques such as Follicular Unit Transplantation (FUT) and Follicular Unit Extraction (FUE) have been developed.

This chapter aims to provide an overview of hair transplant basics and consultation for specialists and plastic surgeons. It will cover the different types of hair transplant techniques. These factors influence the success of the procedure, the preoperative and postoperative care, and the potential risks and complications associated with hair transplant surgery. Additionally, we will discuss the importance of consultation in hair transplant surgery, including the evaluation of the patient's medical history, the examination of the scalp, and the discussion of the patient's expectations and goals.

12.2 Part 1: Basics of Hair Transplant

12.2.1 Section 1: Types of Hair Transplant

Though many causes of hair loss exist, by far the most common aetiology is androgenic alopecia (AGA), an androgen-sensitive pattern of hair loss that affects both men and women.

There are several types of hair transplant techniques, including FUE and FUT. This section will discuss the differences and similarities between these techniques.

Follicular Unit Extraction (FUE) is a minimally invasive hair transplant technique that involves harvesting hair follicles individually from the donor area using a tiny, specialised punch. The extracted follicles are then transplanted into the recipient area. This technique leaves small, circular scars in the donor area, which the surrounding hair can easily conceal. FUE is suitable for patients who have a limited donor area and prefer to keep shorter haircuts.

The major advantage of FUE is that it permits the use of beard and body hair which is essential in advanced cases of baldness with limited scalp donor area [4]. Refer to Table 12.1 for differences between beard and body hair.

Table 12.1 Characteristics of grafts from beard and body area as donor hair

Characteristics	Beard hair as donor	Body hair as donor
Calibre of hair	Coarse and thick	Fine and short
Useful for implantation in	Vertex and mid-front area with scalp hair	Frontal and temporal area with scalp hair
Harvesting technique	Easier	Cumbersome
Extraction process	Faster	Slower
Anagen phase	Longer	Shorter
Tumescence required	Less	More

Body hair lie more superficial in the dermis as compared to scalp hair. They also emerge at a more acute angle from the skin surface in comparison to the scalp hair. Usually, body hair grows singly with 1–2 hair follicles within each follicular unit [5].

12.2.1.1 Beard, Eyebrow and Eyelash Transplant

Hair transplant is also indicated for aesthetic enhancement in patients who desire denser beard, eyebrow, or eyelashes. It can also be performed for reconstruction of beard, eyebrows, and eyelashes in those suffering from alopecia areata (stable), traumatic scars, trichotillomania, acid burns, etc.

Follicular Unit Transplantation (FUT), also known as strip harvesting, involves the removal of a strip of skin from the donor area, which is then dissected under microscope into individual follicular units. The extracted follicles are then transplanted into the recipient area. This technique leaves a linear scar in the donor area, which can be concealed by surrounding hair. FUT is suitable for patients who require a large number of hair follicles.

Regarding differences, FUE is a minimally invasive process that does not require the removal of a strip of skin from the donor location and only grafts are selected and harvested. In contrast, FUT consists of the removal of a strip of skin. Additionally, FUE may result in less scarring compared to FUT.

Currently, FUE represents the more common approach due to its potential advantages over FUT [6], which include:

- Increased number of grafts can be harvested in multiple sessions
- The patient's hairstyle is not a factor since scarring is less apparent
- Donor site laxity and density are not a significant deterrent
- Postoperative pain and healing time are less
- The surgeon can target follicular groups of a specific size or hairs with a specific diameter or pigmentation
- The surgeon can target hairs outside the typical donor site (i.e., parietal scalp, chest, back, beard, pubis) if needed.

On the contrary, FUT may be preferable to FUE [7] given FUT's reported advantages, which include:

- Shorter operative: Though FUE operative time is typically longer than FUT, recent advancements in FUE extraction techniques (e.g., automated mechanical instruments and robotic technology) may close this operative time gap by offering decreased extraction times compared to the traditional, manual FUE techniques
- Less follicular transection rate
- Less of a learning curve
- Can be done without shaving
- Long hair transplant is easier with FUT

The choice of hair transplant technique depends on various factors, including the patient's hair type, the extent of hair loss, the amount of donor hair available, and the patient's preferences. To select the optimal approach for the patient, consulting with a trained and experienced hair transplant surgeon is critical.

12.2.2 Section 2: Procedure of Hair Transplant

In this section, we will discuss the procedure of hair transplant in terms of the following aspects:

- Pre-operative preparations
- Hairline design
- Anaesthesia
- Graft extraction and preparation
- Graft implantation
- Post-operative care

Pre-operative preparations involve evaluating the patient's medical history and performing a physical examination to determine if the patient is a suitable candidate for the procedure. The surgeon will discuss the patient's expectations and goals and provide instructions on pre-operative care, such as avoiding any medications that may increase the risk of bleeding.

Preoperative Checklist [2] include:

1. Stop minoxidil 2 weeks prior to the procedure as it may increase bleeding.
2. Avoid alcohol 2 days before and after the procedure.
3. Preoperative tranquilizer in an anxious patient.
4. Avoiding smoking, NSAIDs at least 7 days prior to the surgery as these may increase bleeding.
5. Preoperative photographs; top, front, side and back views.
6. Informed valid consent.

Preoperative laboratory studies [2] to be performed include Complete blood count including platelet count, bleeding and clotting time (or prothrombin time and activated partial thromboplastin time), blood chemistry profile including sugar, ECG, Antibodies for hepatitis B surface antigen and HIV screening tests may be performed if considered essential.

Hairline design is a critical aspect of the procedure. The surgeon will work with the patient to create a natural-looking hairline that matches the patient's facial features and aesthetic preferences. The hairline design may involve marking the recipient area with a surgical pen or using computer imaging software.

Facial aesthetics influence the art of hairline design which depends on:

- The shape of the face
- Age and gender of the patient—Refer Table 12.2

Table 12.2 Differences between male and female hairline characteristics

Characteristics of Male Hairline	Characteristics of Female Hairline
Mid-frontal point (MFP) is around 7–8 cm. From midpoint of glabella	Normally lower than male hairline with MFP at 5.5–6.5 cm
Temporo-frontal angles are 0.5–1 cm above the MFP and hairline sloping upwards laterally	Temporo-frontal angles are rounded and are at same level as MFP or lower
Temporo-frontal angles are sharply defined	Temporo-frontal angles are ill defined
Temporal point well defined	Temporo-parietal point merging with the hairline
	Widows peak seen often
	Hair at temporo-frontal zone is fine and acutely sloping downwards.

- Profession of the patient
- Number of hair patient has
- Patient's expectations
- It should be designed in an irregularly irregular manner
- Should be futuristic
- Density should be like a forest "single follicles first & multiples behind"

12.2.2.1 Hairline Design Depends on

- Following the existing hair
- The "Rule of Thirds"- balance the facial thirds to follow the golden proportions
- Measurement from the Glabella being at around 7–9 cm.
- Shingle Point- where the steep angle of the forehead meets the flat angle of the scalp.
- Determine the zones- definite (dense hair) and transition (less dense hair) zone—Refer Fig. 12.1
- Make sure hairline has irregularities both macro and micro

Anaesthesia is administered to the patient to ensure comfort during the procedure. Local anaesthesia is typically used in the donor and recipient areas, and the patient remains fully conscious. Two percent lignocaine with adrenaline is generally used for anaesthesia. The upper limit of lignocaine has been accepted around 6–7 mg/kg wt. In addition, injection of tumescent saline solution with epinephrine has been generally, but not universally, recommended. Tumescence has the advantage that it produces vasoconstriction and reduces intraoperative bleeding. It also lifts the subcutis from the underlying vessels and prevents damage to large vessels and nerves [8].

Graft extraction and preparation involves harvesting the hair follicles from the donor area. The surgeon may use FUE or FUT methods to extract the grafts. In the strip or FUT method, grafts are sliced from the strip of skin and further slivered under microscope. Whereas, in FUE method, follicles are directly harvested from the skin with the help of motor or manual punches. The harvested grafts are then carefully separated and prepared for implantation.

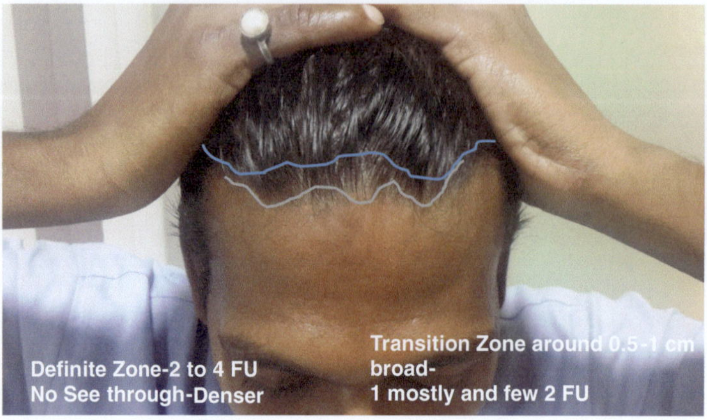

Fig. 12.1 Demarcation of transition zone (white line) and the denser definite zone (blue line) for replication of natural hairline and gradual density of hair pattern

12.2.2.2 Theory of Safe Donor Zone in FUE [9]

The theory of "safe donor zone" is particularly important in today's era of hair transplant surgery where most of our patients present to us with advanced grades of alopecia with a limited donor area. Due to a limited donor area from the scalp and beard, most surgeons find it difficult to determine the "safe donor area" available for graft harvesting. "Safe donor zone" is defined as an area in which progression of permanent hair loss does not occur.

Reasons for graft desiccation is due to dehydration, transection, blunt trauma, and ischemia reperfusion injury. Reducing the duration between graft extraction and implantation is crucial to improve graft survival. Normal saline, ringer lactate, hypothermosol A, ATP activated liposomal solution, and platelet rich plasma are some of the commonly used holding situations [10].

Graft implantation involves transplanting the harvested follicles into the recipient area. The surgeon will make tiny incisions in the scalp to create the recipient sites. The grafts are implanted into the recipient sites using forceps or a specialized tool called implanters. Implanters are pen like devices with a sharp needle at the end tip which loads the grafts and inserts it into the scalp skin. With implanters there is no need to make the pre-holes, thus making it a one-step implantation method with obvious advantages such as uniform graft depth placement, faster implantation, lesser bleeding and reduced trauma to the grafts.

12.2.2.3 Principles of Implantation

- Maximise visualisation during placement
- Use magnification
- Keep your eye on the target

- Follow a pattern
- Control bleeding
- Avoid dehydration and desiccation
- Ensure proper graft sizing
- Control incision spacing and depth

The grafts are inserted into the recipient slits using fine-angled forceps. It is important to place the grafts in an atraumatic technique. In FUT, the follicular units (FUs) are grasped by subcutaneous tissue below the hair bulbs to place them into the recipient slits. In FUE, it is advised to follow a "No root touch" technique where the FUs are held by the upper third without damaging the bulb. A steady pressure is applied to ensure that the grafts are at the level of the surrounding skin. Burying the grafts beneath the level of the skin must be avoided otherwise it can give a pitted appearance leading to epidermal cysts. A cobblestone appearance is seen if the grafts are too elevated from the surface [11]. The techniques for graft insertion are as follows:

(a) The "stick and place method" involves creating a recipient slit, followed by insertion of hairs into the site by an assistant immediately.
(b) Creating all the recipient sites at one time and then placing the grafts one by one.
(c) Using implanters which involves the use of pre-loaded pen-like instruments with an extracted graft in its hollow end, directly into the scalp.
(d) Creating all the recipient sites and then using an implanter to insert all the grafts together.

12.2.3 *Implantation Techniques: (Refer Table 12.3)*

1. Pre-hole making:
   (a) 1 Person Pre-Hole: Incisions are made and the follicular unit is inserted using forceps by the surgeon

Table 12.3 Comparison of various techniques for graft placement used in follicular unit extraction [12]

Serial no.	Characteristics	Stick and place method	Premade recipient sites	Implanter
1.	Performed by	Physician	Physician and assistant	Physician
2.	Mechanical graft handling	Present	Present (one-hand technique)	Very less
			Absent (two-hand technique)	
3.	Popping risk	High	Less	High
4.	Learning curve	High	High	Less
5.	Cost	Less	Less	High
6.	Position of patient's head	Supine	Supine	Supine

   (b) 2 Person Pre-Hole: Incisions are made and the follicular units are inserted by one surgeon while the assistant facilitates placement by holding the slits wide

      - Less traumatic and easier graft insertion
      - Helpful in difficult cases in which the patients are experiencing above average bleeding or graft popping

2. Stick & Place:

   (a) Slits are filled with a hair graft immediately after they are made
   (b) Less risk of leaving openings unfilled or inadvertently placing two grafts into the same opening
   (c) Easier to identify and follow the exact angle and direction of incision
   (d) Greater demand on surgeon's time
   (e) Only one team placing at a time
   (f) Long learning curve to achieve speed
   (g) Less control over pattern and distribution

3. Use of Implanters

Post-operative care is crucial in ensuring optimal recovery, excellent results and minimizing complications. The patient will receive instructions on how to care for the surgical donor and recipient sites, including washing and grooming. The patient may be prescribed medications to manage pain, swelling, and the risk of infection. It is essential to avoid strenuous activities and exposure to direct sunlight during the recovery period.

CPP is an algorithmic model devised by Dr. Viral Desai for ease of treatment planning a hair transplant case (Refer Fig. 12.2). The protocol helps one plan a surgery based on artistic aspects, mathematical aspects, psychosocial and medical parameters in a methodical manner to avoid missing out on any crucial aspects. To perform hair restoration surgery in a very precise and accurate way, one should have a good grasp of the **mathematical** aspects and apply them to the **science** of surgery in an **artistic** way in order to achieve natural, excellent and successful results every single time.

12.2.4 Comprehensive Procedure Protocol

1. **Medical evaluation**

   (a) Review medical history
   (b) Thorough systemic examination
   (c) Local anaesthesia suitability
   (d) Check for any medical disorders including allergies

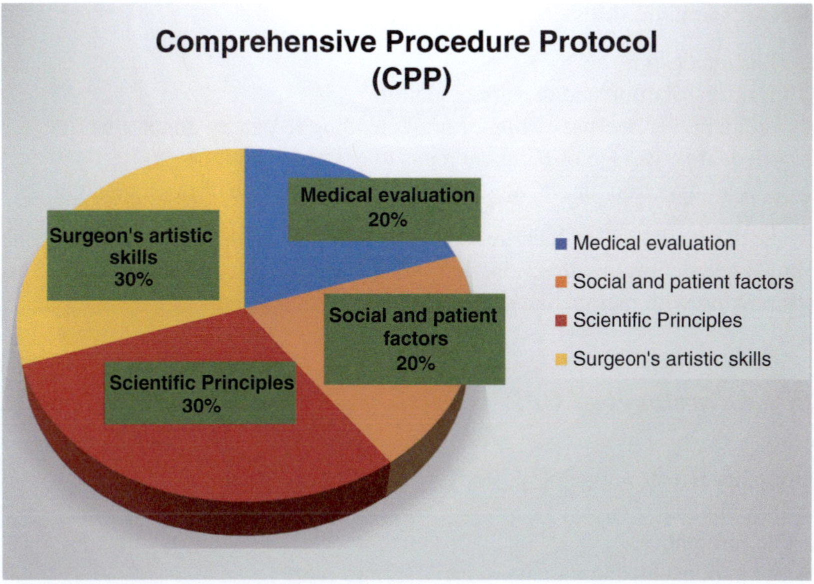

Fig. 12.2 Comprehensive Procedure Protocol (CPP)

2. **Social and patient factors**
    (a) Patient query form
    (b) Patient's requirements and expectations
    (c) Varied treatment options
    (d) Thorough understanding of all types of treatments
    (e) Type of treatment selection by patient
    (f) Patient photographs and informed consent
3. **Scientific Principles**
    (a) Alopecia testing tools
    (b) Planning and timing of sessions
    (c) Donor area evaluation
    (d) Safe donor area calculation
    (e) Estimation of number of extractable grafts
    (f) Recipient area calibration
    (g) Recipient area gradation of grafts from hairline to centre to crown
    (h) Graft distribution and density planning to achieve best cosmetic natural results
    (i) Total number of grafts that can be transplanted in a lifetime

4. **Surgeon's artistic skills**
   (a) Hairline design
   (b) Graft distribution and density gradation
   (c) Avoidance of overharvesting of grafts leading to patchy donor area
   (d) Adequate coverage of recipient areas to get a natural look
   (e) Correct direction, depth, angle and emergence profile of implanted grafts

Pillars and cornerstones of hair treatment planning involve concepts of hairline designing, zone definition, direction, density, distribution also should take into consideration along with factors like profession, ethnicity, age, etc.

12.2.5 Advantages of CPP

1. Comprehensive coverage of all steps included for treatment planning
2. Easily replicable model
3. Easy to remember
4. Greater patient satisfaction and reduced failure rates

CPP can be thus kept in mind while devising critical steps of the surgery such as graft distribution, density and hairline planning which should strike a delicate balance between art and science as well as satisfying patient requirements.

12.2.6 Section 3: Benefits and Risks of Hair Transplant

- Benefits of hair transplant
- Possible risks and complications

12.2.6.1 Benefits of Hair Transplant

Improved Appearance: Hair transplant surgery can help patients restore their hairline and achieve a more youthful and aesthetically pleasing appearance. The procedure can also help to fill in bald patches and improve the overall density of hair.

Long-Lasting Results: Hair transplant surgery can provide long-lasting results, as the transplanted hair follicles are taken from areas of the scalp that are genetically resistant to balding. This means the transplanted hair will be unlikely to fall out or thin over time.

Low Maintenance: Once the transplanted hair has fully grown, it can be treated and styled like natural hair. Patients can wash, cut, and style their hair without special care or maintenance requirements.

Self-Esteem Boost: Hair loss can significantly impact a person's self-esteem and confidence. Hair transplant surgery can help patients feel more confident and self-assured by restoring their hairline and improving their appearance.

12.2.6.2 Possible Risks and Complications

Infection: As with any surgical procedure, there is a risk of infection after hair transplant surgery. Patients should take proper care of their scalp after the process and follow all post-operative instructions their surgeon provides.

Bleeding: Hair transplant surgery can cause bleeding, particularly during harvesting donor hair follicles. However, this is generally a minor issue and can be easily controlled by the surgeon.

Scarring: Hair transplant surgery can cause scarring at both the donor and recipient sites. However, skilled surgeons can minimize scarring by using advanced techniques and minimizing trauma to the scalp.

Pain and Discomfort: Patients may experience some discomfort after hair transplant surgery. Pain and Discomfort can usually be managed with over-the-counter pain medications.

Swelling: Some patients may experience swelling in the forehead or around the eyes after hair transplant surgery. This is generally a temporary side effect and will resolve independently over time.

Itching and Tingling: Patients may experience itching and tingling in the scalp for several weeks after hair transplant surgery. This is a normal healing process and will subside over time.

Aesthetic: Improper hairline, uneven grafts distribution, patchy hair restoration.

12.3 Part 2: Consultation

12.3.1 Section 1: Purpose of Consultation

- Importance of consultation
- What to expect from a consultation

A consultation for hair transplant is a crucial step in the treatment process, as it provides an opportunity for the treating doctor to evaluate the patient's candidacy for the procedure, discuss the potential benefits and risks, and develop an individualised treatment plan that meets the patient's goals and expectations.

12.3.1.1 Importance of Consultation for Hair Transplant by a Specialist

There are three primary purposes for consultation. The first is to provide information to the prospective patient; the second is to establish the compatibility of the patient and doctor; and the third is to set realistic, practical, and wise goals both in the short term and, more importantly, in a long time.

A doctor's consultation for a hair transplant is essential to ensure that the patient is a suitable candidate for the procedure. The specialist will evaluate the patient's hair loss pattern, density, and overall health status to determine whether he/she is fit for the procedure. Further, they will also discuss the patient's expectations and goals, which can help to develop a realistic treatment plan that meets the patient's needs.

A specialist's consultation for a hair transplant involves several essential components for ensuring a successful outcome. These components include:

12.3.1.2 Patient Selection

- Very few general physical disorders contraindicate hair transplant, provided they can be brought under reasonable medical control.
- Hypertension, for example, can cause excessive bleeding during and after operations, resulting in poor graft acceptance, but once hypertension is under control, these patients present no further difficulties.
- Even patients with moderate cardiac disease or previous cardiac bypass operations can undergo the procedure if it is adequately staged with smaller than usual sessions, provided epinephrine is used cautiously.
- Diabetic patients should probably have sessions spread at least six months apart because of their impaired peripheral blood supply and the increased permeability of their vasculature. The latter causes increased postoperative tissue oedema, further decreasing circulation.
- Local cutaneous disorders that could prevent success, such as active cutaneous lupus erythematosus, alopecia areata, and severe folliculitis, are contraindications for surgery.
- In addition, a consultation with a specialist can be particularly beneficial for patients with underlying skin or scalp conditions, such as dandruff, psoriasis or eczema.
- The specialist can evaluate the patient's skin and scalp health and recommend any necessary treatments to ensure that the patient's skin is healthy and prepared for the hair transplant procedure.

Transplanting should not be carried out until treatment has controlled these diseases and until they have been quiescent for at least 6–12 months.

12.3.1.3 How to Manage Unhappy or Difficult Patients

There are several patient characteristics [13] that have been cited as contributing factors to certain clinical challenging interactions include the following:

- Unrealistic expectations.
- Ignoring medical advice.
- Apparent dissatisfaction in care.

- Persistent complaints despite efforts to help.
- Insistence on being prescribed unnecessary drugs.
- Being verbally abusive and disrespectful.

In addition to these problematic personality categories, there may be other types of patients such as rude patients and know-it-all patients. These patients present a challenge to the surgeon, who should consider aligning the patients' expectations with the expected outcome of the hair transplant surgery as a sine qua non to admitting the patient under their care [14].

12.3.1.4 What to Expect from a Consultation for Hair Transplant by a Specialist

During a specialist's consultation for a hair transplant, patients can expect to undergo a comprehensive evaluation of their scalp and hair health. The specialist will evaluate the patient's hair loss pattern, density, and overall hair health to determine the best course of action for the patient.

The specialist will also review the patient's medical history and ask questions about any underlying health conditions or medications that may affect the procedure. The specialist may also take photographs of the patient's scalp and hair to document the extent of the hair loss and track the progress of the process.

During the consultation, the specialist will discuss the potential risks and benefits of the procedure and answer any questions or concerns the patient may have. The specialist will also develop an individualised treatment plan tailored to the patient's needs and goals, which may include discussing the different hair transplant techniques available, such as FUT or FUE, and determining which approach is most appropriate for the patient's needs.

Overall, a specialist's consultation for a hair transplant is an essential step in the treatment process, as it can help patients make an informed decision about whether the procedure is right for them and can ensure that they receive the best possible outcome.

12.3.2 Section 2: Components of Consultation

- Medical history
- Hair loss evaluation
- Hair restoration goals and expectations
- Discussion of hair transplant options
- Post-operative care and follow-up

Medical History: The specialist will review the patient's medical history in depth to identify any underlying health conditions or medications that may affect the hair transplant procedure. The specialist will also ask questions about the patient's family history of hair loss and any previous hair loss treatments the patient may have undergone. Use a questionnaire that elicits information about the patient's general medical history and history of hair loss.

You can ask if the patient has a history of:

- Bleeding problems (nose bleeds, gum bleeds, easy bruising, etc.)
- Poor or abnormal healing (wide scars, raised scars, larger scars, keloids, slow healing)
- Liver problems (Hepatitis)
- Hypertension
- Heart disease (heart attack, arrhythmia, or irregular pulse, heart murmur, etc.)
- Lung disease (asthma, pneumonia, chronic bronchitis)
- Hormonal disorders (Diabetes, Thyroid problems, etc.)
- Kidney, Bladder disease (prostate)
- Stomach disease (ulcers, heartburn, etc.)
- Neurologic disease (stroke, seizure, fainting)
- Hay fever, Hives, Eczema or seasonal allergies
- Glaucoma
- Any artificial prostheses, artificial heart valves, metal pins
- Disorders of the Immune system
- Tattoos
- Blood transfusions
- Emotional problems (depression, anxiety, panic disorder, etc.)
- Rare Disorders (Hereditary Angioedema, Malignant Hyperthermia)
- Smoking, alcohol intake
- Are you allergic to any of the following local anaesthetics and other medications which are occasionally used in surgery:
  - Novocaine
  - Xylocaine
  - Skin Tape
  - Iodine
  - Valium
  - Penicillin
  - Codeine
  - Prednisone
  - Substances applied to skin
- List all prescription or non-prescription medications, drugs, vitamins or nutritional supplements you take either regularly or occasionally: (Including Rogaine, Vitamin E, over-the-counter pain and arthritis medications).
- Please list any operations, or serious medical illness not mentioned above

Hair Loss Evaluation: The specialist will evaluate the patient's hair loss pattern, density, and overall hair health to determine the extent of the hair loss and the best course of action for the patient. This may involve a physical examination of the scalp and hair and a review of any diagnostic tests, such as blood tests or scalp biopsies.

The hair is then examined, and the colour, texture, calibre, curl, and density are noted in the chart. This is also recorded if particular areas are relatively sparse, e.g., the temporal region. The eventual sizes of the donor and recipient areas are estimated after careful examination.

Sometimes, the hair is wetted to aid in this estimation, conducted under a bright light. The less experienced the physician, the wiser it is to soak the hair.

Scalp dermoscopy or `trichoscopy' is an invaluable tool for every specialist. It is a noninvasive technique for the evaluation of patients with hair loss that allows for magnified visualization of the hair and scalp skin. It may be performed with a manual dermoscope (×10 magnification) or a videodermoscope (up to ×1000 magnification). In particular, trichoscopy enhances the diagnosis of androgenetic alopecia, alopecia areata, telogen effluvium, trichotillomania, congenital triangular alopecia, scarring alopecia, tinea capitis and hair shaft disorders [15]. This method is simple, quick and easy to perform, reduces the need for scalp biopsy, is well accepted by patients, and is useful for monitoring treatment and follow-up.

Trichoscopy has been widely used as a diagnostic as well as a prognostic tool to measure anisotrichosis in cases of overt androgenetic alopecia and female pattern hair loss (FPHL) and to distinguish them from telogen effluvium [16]. It can be used to distinguish FPHL from diffuse and subtotal alopecia areata (AA) as well as trichotillomania from AA which can have similar clinical presentations. Trichoscopy also helps in monitoring treatment response in patients of AA.

The donor area follicular unit (FU) density, hair density, and hair thickness are the most important parameters to be evaluated (using a micrometer). Patients with normal-to-high FU density (>65 FU/cm^2) and thick hair (50–60 μ) are considered good candidates while patients with diffuse hair loss, low FU density (40–50 FUs/cm^2), and donor hair miniaturization (20% miniaturized) are poor candidates [17]. Coarse hair and curly hair will have better coverage compared to fine hair and straight hair.

Currently, the **Hamilton-Norwood classification system for males** (Refer Figs. 12.3 and 12.4) and **the Ludwig system for females** (Refer Fig. 12.5) are most commonly used to describe patterns of hair loss [18].

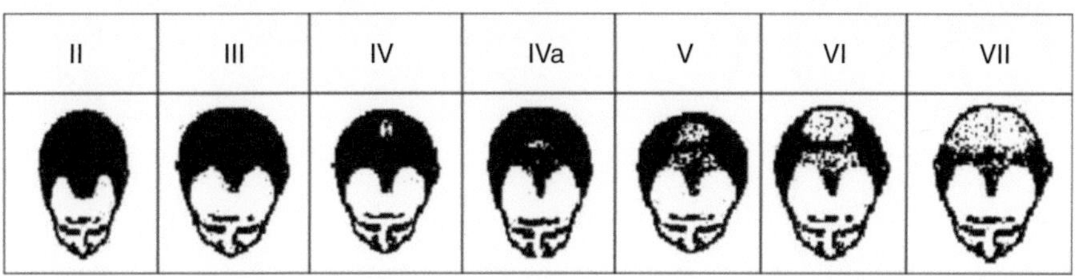

Fig. 12.3 Hamilton-Norwood classification system for males

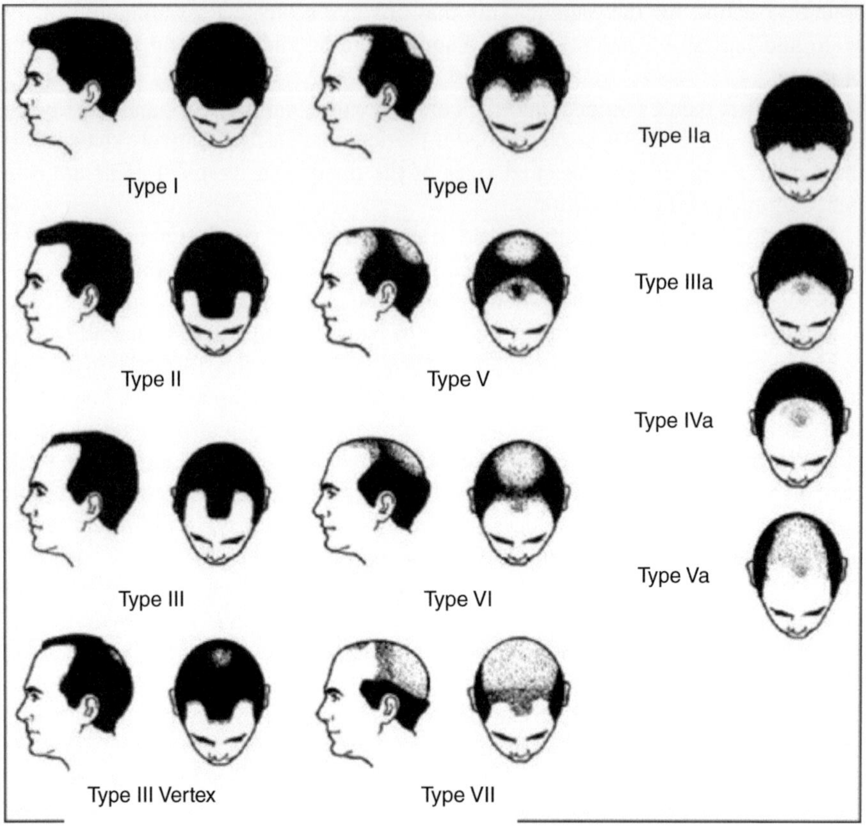

Fig. 12.4 Hamilton-Norwood classification system for males

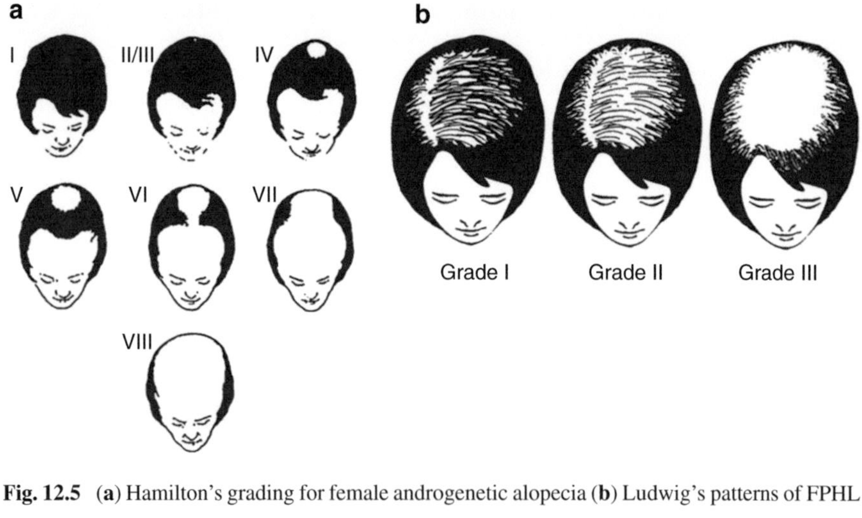

Fig. 12.5 (**a**) Hamilton's grading for female androgenetic alopecia (**b**) Ludwig's patterns of FPHL

A copy of Norwood's schematic classification of alopecia may also be added to the chart and used to record the family history and estimated ultimate prognosis in a male patient.

12.3.2.1 Hamilton-Norwood Classification

Type I: There is minimal or no recession of the hairline.

Type II: There are triangular, usually symmetrical, areas of recession at the frontotemporal hairline.

Type III: This represents the minimal extent of hair loss sufficient to be considered as baldness according to Norwood. There is deep symmetrical recession at the temples that are bare or only sparsely covered by hair. In Type III vertex, the hair loss is primarily from the vertex with limited recession of the frontotemporal hairline that does not exceed the degree of recession seen in Type III.

Type IV: The frontotemporal recession is more severe than in Type III and there is sparse hair or no hair on the vertex. The two areas of hair loss are separated by a band of moderately dense hair that extends across the top. This band connects with the fully haired fringe on the sides of the scalp.

Type V: The vertex hair loss region is still separated from the frontotemporal region but it is less distinct. The band of hair across the crown is narrower and sparser and the vertex and frontotemporal regions of hair loss are bigger.

Type VI: The bridge of hair that crosses the crown is gone with only sparse hair remaining. The frontotemporal and vertex regions are joined together and the extent of hair loss is greater.

Type VII: The most severe form of hair loss and only a narrow band of hair in a horseshoe shape remains on the sides and back of the scalp. This hair is usually not dense and may be quite fine.

Norwood also defined a Type A variant from his standard classification system, which is distinguished by two major features and two minor features.

The major features are: (1) the anterior border of the hairline progresses to the rear without leaving an island of hair in the mid-frontal region and (2) there is no simultaneous development of a bald area on the vertex. Instead, the frontal hairline recession keeps progressing to the rear of the scalp.

The minor features are: (1) there is a persistent sparse hair scattering in the area of hair loss and (2) the horseshoe-shaped fringe areas of hair that remain on the side and back of the scalp tend to be wider and reach higher on the head compared to Norwood's standard. The various Type A variants described by Norwood are as follows:

Type IIA: The hairline is anterior to the coronal plane 2 cm anterior to the external auditory meatus.

Type IIIA: The hairline has receded back to a point between the limit of Type IIA and the level of the external auditory meatus.

Type IVA: The hairline has receded beyond the external auditory meatus but has not reached the vertex.

Type VA: The area of denudation includes the vertex. Hair loss more severe than Type VA cannot be distinguished from Types VI or VII.

Norwood classification is one of the most detailed classification systems for male patterned hair loss and is the most widely used classification worldwide but is too detailed, divided, and complicated to be used for various surgical operations. Moreover, it also does not list some peculiar types of baldness (a balding patch on the vertex or occiput with a preserved anterior hairline) and is not very helpful in determining the surgical method. Numerous researchers proposed newer classification systems keeping the simplicity of classification and surgical aspects of treatment in mind.

For female patients, Hamilton's and Ludwig's schematic drawings may also be utilized:

Hair Restoration Goals and Expectations: The specialist will discuss the patient's hair restoration goals and expectations to develop a treatment plan that meets the patient's needs. This may include discussing the desired hairline, density, and overall appearance of the hair after the procedure.

It is also important to establish realistic goals for each patient. Young patients, for example, may want to reproduce teenage level and shaped hairlines, and it is obviously advantageous to advise them that what they should really be deciding on is a hairline that will be appropriate for them at any age, including their fifties, sixties, and seventies.

The term megasession refers to transplanting greater than 3000 follicular unit grafts in a single day procedure [19]. By transplanting a large number of grafts, megasessions are capable of definitively treating a significant area of the scalp in a single session. Patients must be carefully selected to determine whether they are appropriate candidates for an extended procedure. FUE megasession has the advantages of decreased frequency of repeat surgery and patients with severe AGA are encouraged toward this hair restoration treatment [20].

A compromise should be sought between what they would ideally like at their present age and what will look appropriate when they are much older. In addition, they should be advised of the likely eventual extent of the area of Male Pattern Baldness and the corresponding size of the potential donor area, as well as the probable ultimate hair density of the donor area (especially in the temporal area).

To set realistic goals and avoid unhappy patients following steps can be taken [14]:

- Predict future hair loss
- Hair style to create better illusion of density
- Continuation of medical management
- Explain: combined medical and hair transplant gives best results
- Multiple sessions may be needed

12.3.2.2 During the Consultation

- Realistic expectation
- Address areas of most concern

- Number and layout of grafts
- Number of sessions required
- Possible density

12.3.2.3 During the Pre-Operative Stage

- It is the role of the surgeon to counsel the patient, set right their expectations, and obtain informed consent at this stage. The "BATHE" technique [21] (Refer Fig. 12.6) is a psychotherapeutic screening test for anxiety, depression, and situational stress disorders procedure. It comprises four specific questions, each followed by an empathic response.
- In addition to the BATHE technique, the surgeon should be aware of the patient's appearance and conduct. The indicators of a problematic personality of patient must be observed and documented [14].

12.3.2.4 During the Surgery (Refer Fig. 12.7)

- Pleasant experience
- Light music
- Careful talking among team
- Pain management
- During the operative stage, patients may develop judgments regarding the surgeon's capabilities and the environment of the clinic in general.
- It may be advisable to have a standard operating procedure for the operative stage to ensure that the patient does not feel biased against owing to any deviation of the conduct of the clinical staff regarding one patient versus another [14].
- A recent publication proposed the use of the ROAR [22] (reflective, objective, assessment, reassurance) approach to moderate a difficult patient interaction (Refer Fig. 12.8).

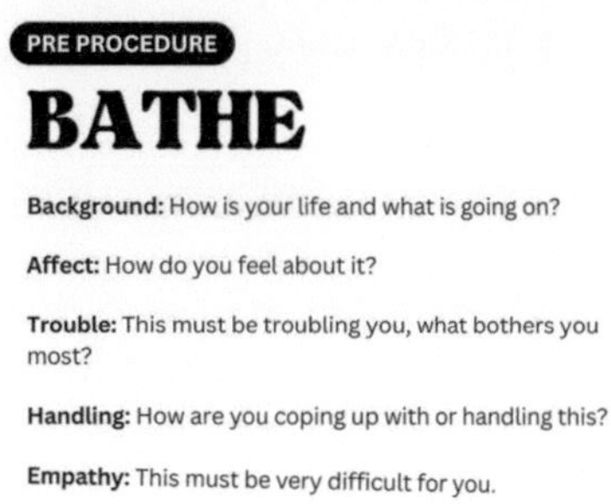

Fig. 12.6 BATHE Technique

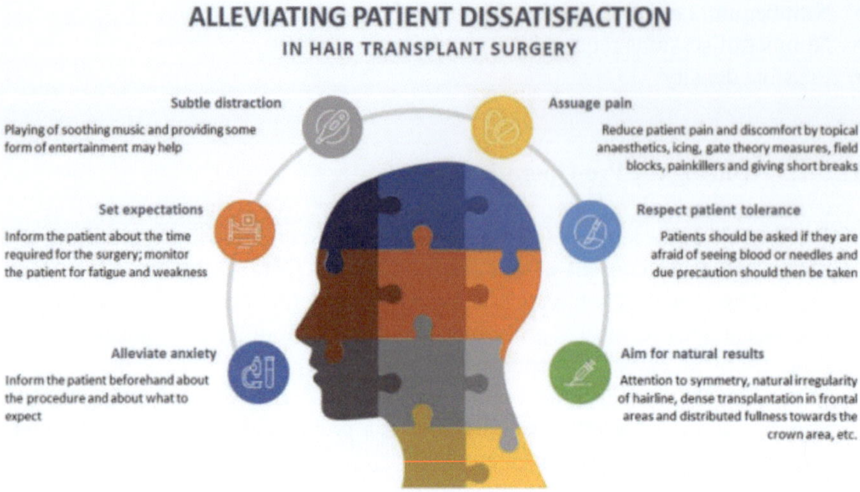

Fig. 12.7 Standard Operating Procedure Framework

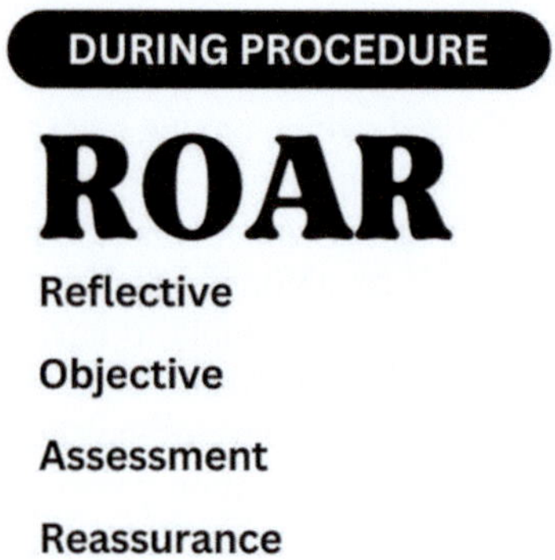

Fig. 12.8 ROAR Approach

- ROAR involves reflecting the patient's distress, engaging the patient in the objective evaluation, providing an acknowledgment of the uncertain aspects of the plan of care, and providing the required reassurance to the patient.

12.3.2.5 In the Post-Operative Stage

- After a hair transplant surgery, a common factor that causes discontentment among patients is dissatisfaction with the results.
- Many patients who may be cooperative during the surgery may turn hostile if the expected results are not achieved or complications arise.
- The "BLAST" technique (Refer Fig. 12.9) is a complaint-resolution method that is useful for patient care and as a clinical teaching tool [23].

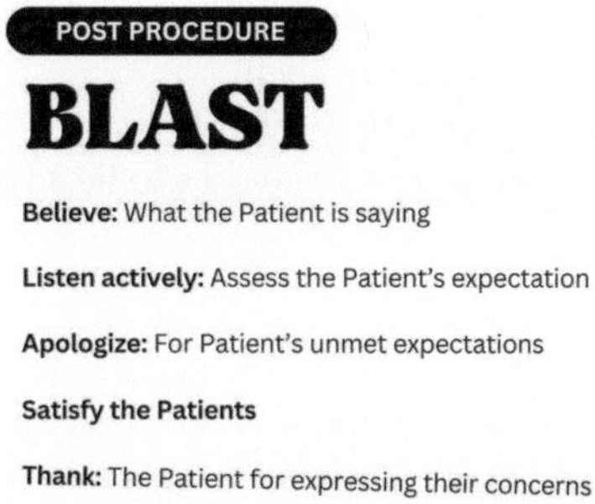
POST PROCEDURE
BLAST
Believe: What the Patient is saying
Listen actively: Assess the Patient's expectation
Apologize: For Patient's unmet expectations
Satisfy the Patients
Thank: The Patient for expressing their concerns

Fig. 12.9 BLAST Technique

Objectives should be matched to these indispensable factors and should be based on the worst possible scenario that can be realistically foreseen in the long run for that individual.

12.3.2.6 Summary Points to Be Followed for Better Consultation

Points to be explained:

- Predict future hair loss
- Hair style to create better illusion of density
- Continuation of medical management
- Explain: combined medical and surgical treatment gives best results
- Multiple sessions may be needed

During the consultation

- Realistic expectation
- Areas of most concern
- Number and layout of grafts
- Number of sessions required
- Possible density
- Best possible outcome
- Cost of procedure
- Use of body hair
- Evaluation of body dysmorphic disorder

During the surgery

- Pleasant experience
- Light music

- Careful talking among team
- Pain management
- Inform every step
- Show grafts and area to be covered
- No criticism and discussion

Discussion of Hair Transplant Options: The specialist will discuss the different hair transplant options available, such FUT or FUE, and determine which technique is most appropriate for the patient's needs. The treating doctor will also explain the procedure in detail, including the potential risks and benefits, the expected outcomes, and the recovery process.

Post-operative Care and Follow-Up: The specialist will provide the patient with detailed instructions for post-operative care, including how to care for the scalp and hair after the procedure and any medications that may be necessary. The specialist will also schedule follow-up appointments to monitor the patient's progress and ensure that the patient is healing properly.

In summary, consultation for a hair transplant is a comprehensive evaluation involving a thorough medical history review, hair loss evaluation, discussion of hair restoration goals and expectations, explanation of hair transplant options, and detailed instructions for post-operative care and follow-up. By addressing each component, the specialist can develop an individualised treatment plan that meets the patient's needs and ensures the best possible outcome.

In conclusion, a hair transplant is a surgical procedure that involves placing hair follicles from the donor area to the recipient area. The process involves important steps such as pre-operative preparations, hairline design, anaesthesia, graft extraction and preparation, implantation, and post-operative care. The procedure's success depends on several factors, including the surgeon's experience and skill, the patient's suitability, and adherence to pre-operative and post-operative instructions. Patients should consult with a qualified and experienced hair transplant surgeon to determine if a hair transplant is suitable for their specific case.

References

1. Bernstein RM, Rassman WR, Seager D, Shapiro R, et al. Standardizing the classification and description of follicular unit transplantation and mini-micro grafting techniques. Dermatologic Surg. 1998;24:957–63.
2. Patwardhan N, Mysore V. Hair transplantation: standard guidelines of care. Indian J Dermatol Venereol Leprol. 2008;74:46–53.
3. Shiell RC. A review of modern surgical hair restoration techniques. J Cutan Aesthet Surg. 2008;1(1):12–6. https://doi.org/10.4103/0974-2077.41150. PMID: 20300332; PMCID: PMC2840892.
4. Chouhan K, Roga G, Kumar A, Gupta J. Approach to hair transplantation in advanced grade baldness by follicular unit extraction: a retrospective analysis of 820 cases. J Cutan Aesthet Surg. 2019;12:215.
5. Paus R, Cotsarelis G. The biology of hair follicles. New Eng J Med. 1999;341:491–7.

6. Gupta AK, Lyons DC, Daigle D. Progression of surgical hair restoration techniques. J Cutan Med Surg. 2015;19(1):17–21.
7. Zito PM, Raggio BS. Hair transplantation, StatPearls [Internet]. Treasure Island: StatPearls [Internet].
8. Seager DJ, Simmons C. Local anesthesia in hair transplantation. Dermatologic Surg. 2002;28:320–8.
9. Chouhan K, Roga G. Hair transplantation in androgenetic alopecia. Cosmoderma. 2021;1:20.
10. Kim JC, Hwang SJ, Lee JJ, Oh BM, Lee SJ, Kim DW, Kim MK. The effects of dehydration, preservation temperature and time on the hair grafts. Ann Dermatol. 2002;14:149–52.
11. Khanna M. Hair transplantation surgery. Indian J Plast Surg. 2008;41:S56.
12. Bansal A, Sethi P, Kumar A, Sahoo AK, Das P. Use of implanters in premade recipient sites for hair transplantation. J Cutan Aesthet Surg. 2019;12(4):250–4. https://doi.org/10.4103/JCAS.JCAS_33_19. PMID: 32001973; PMCID: PMC6967169.
13. Hull SK, Broquet K. How to manage difficult patient encounters. Fam Pract Manag. 2007;14(06):30–4.
14. Desai V. Managing an unhappy patient. Indian J Plast Surg. 2021;54(4):495–500. https://doi.org/10.1055/s-0041-1739249. PMID: 34984091; PMCID: PMC8719954.
15. Lacarrubba F, Micali G, Tosti A. Scalp dermoscopy or trichoscopy. Curr Probl Dermatol. 2015;47:21–32. https://doi.org/10.1159/000369402. Epub 2015 Feb 20.
16. Dhurat RS. Utility of trichoscopy. Indian J Dermatopathol Diagn Dermatol. 2018;5:89–96.
17. Jimenez F, Alam M, Vogel JE, Avram M. Hair transplantation: basic overview. J Am Acad Dermatol. 2021;85:803–14.
18. Gupta M, Mysore V. Classifications of patterned hair loss: a review. J Cutan Aesthet Surg. 2016;9(1):3–12. https://doi.org/10.4103/0974-2077.178536. PMID: 27081243; PMCID: PMC4812885
19. Gabel S. Megasessions: surgical indications and technical perspectives. Facial Plast Surg Clin North Am. 2013;21(3):419–30. https://doi.org/10.1016/j.fsc.2013.06.002.
20. Li KT, Qu Q, Fan ZX, Wang J, Liu F, Hu ZQ, et al. Clinical experience on follicular unit extraction megasession for severe androgenetic alopecia. J Cosmet Dermatol. 2020;19:1481–6.
21. Lieberman JA III, Stuart MR. The BATHE method: incorporating counseling and psychotherapy into the everyday management of patients. Prim Care Companion J Clin Psychiatry. 1999;1(02):35–8.
22. McCarthy JG, Cheatham JG, Singla M. How to approach difficult patient encounters. ROAR Gastroenterology. 2018;155(02):258–61.
23. Steinman HK. A method for working with displeased patientsblast. J Clin Aesthet Dermatol. 2013;6(03):25–8.

Chapter 13
Importance of Nutrition & Diet in PCOS

Nidhi Singh Tandon

13.1 Introduction

PCOS (polycystic ovarian syndrome) is one of the most common female endocrinopathies affecting 15–18% of women of reproductive age [1] and is commonly associated with obesity, menstrual irregularity, infertility, insulin resistance and clinical hyperandrogenism and/or hyperandrogenemia.

Patients with PCOS are at increased risk of obesity, metabolic dysfunction, malignancy, reproductive complications and mood disorders [2].

13.1.1 Physiological Basis

Main causes of physiological basis of PCOS include.

Disorders of gonadotropin hormonal synthesis.

Insulin resistance.

Influence of excessive body fat.

Metabolic pathways involved in PCOS [3].

N. S. Tandon (✉)
Skin Art Clinic, Lucknow, India

R. Singh, N. Sharma (eds.), *A Guide to Hormonal Dermatology*,
https://doi.org/10.1007/978-981-99-7715-4_13

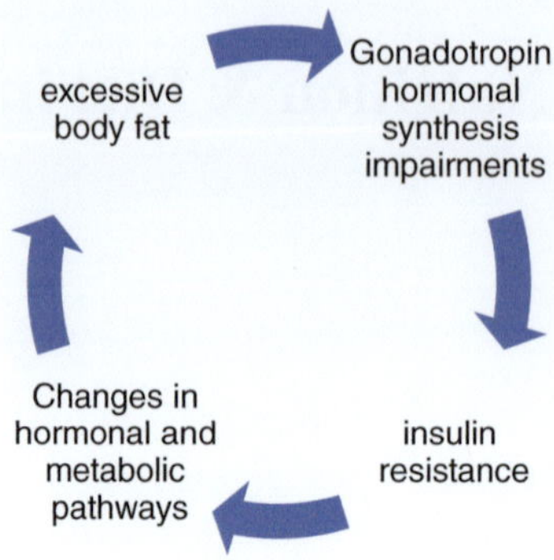

Appropriate functioning and maturation of the ovarian follicle depends on three main organs.

Hypothalamus, pituitary gland and ovaries.

The regulation of hormones in the hypothalamic-pituitary-ovarian system takes place through the axis of negative feedback. Hypothalamus releases GnRH into the pituitary portal circulation. Type of GnRH released is determined by the frequency of the rhythm of the hormone secreted in pulsatile manner called as gonadoliberin. A Low frequency of gonadoliberin results in secretion of follicle stimulating hormone (FSH), while high frequency results in secretion of luteinizing hormone (LH) from the anterior lobe of the pituitary gland. LH causes luteinization of the corpus luteum which then produces testosterone and FSH in turn causes maturation of ovarian follicles and secretion of estrogen into the granulosa cells of ovarian follicles.

When the concentration of luteinizing hormone (LH) increases relatively to FSH, excessive androgen production occurs, which is more common in women with PCOS [4].

Insulin plays an important role in PCOS both directly and indirectly. It acts synergistically with LH to increase production of androgens (theca cells) and reduces the synthesis of SHBG (sex hormone binding globulin) in liver which is a testosterone binding protein.

This results in testosterone circulating in unbound active form [4].

Excess body fat also plays an important role in development of PCOS. Adipose tissue cells produce certain hormones like leptin and resistin that affects functioning of the hypothalamic pituitary-ovary axis by modifying secretion of GnRH, LH, FSH [5]. Leptin is a signal for the hypothalamus to release LH, causing secretion of pituitary GnRH as well. This results in excess androgen synthesis. Adipose tissues also produce inflammatory cytokines that leads to inflammation in PCOS. Excess adipose tissue, increased free radicals due to hyperglycemia and androgens result in development of chronic inflammation in PCOS [4].

Various studies indicate that women with PCOS have higher intake of calories and saturated fat and inadequate fiber consumption in their diet.

Clinical symptoms and risk of chronic diseases in PCOS patients can be exacerbated by alterations in diet.

Szczuko et al. analyzed the diet of 54 women of childbearing age with PCOS and concluded that metabolic disorders related to improper ovarian function are due to unhealthy diets in women with PCOS [6].

13.2 Role of Gut Microbiome

Tremellen and Pearce proposed microbiological hypothesis suggesting that a poor diet leads to dysbiosis of gut microbiota leading to PCOS [7].

The microbiota through its metabolites has complex effect on appetite, lipids and carbohydrate metabolism and may affect body weight too [8, 9].

The gut microbiota can regulate 10% of the hosts genes involved in immune response, proliferation and metabolism [10].

The growth of Bifidobacterium regulates insulin resistance and helps reduce inflammation. Short chain fatty acids (SCFAs) such as acetate and butyrate produced by our gut microflora has influence on glycemia through intestinal hormones like glucagon like peptide (GLP-1) and pancreatic polypeptide (PPY) [11].

The PPY hormone acts as a paracrine substance to stimulate hunger or feeling of satiety in the control center [12].

13.2.1 Oxidative Stress and Chronic Inflammation

Epidemiological studies and large clinical trials have identified low grade chronic inflammation and pro-inflammatory and anti-inflammatory components in diets associated with pathogenesis of PCOS.

Increase in ROS generation and circulating thiobarbituric acid-reactive substances (TBARS) occur in PCOS in response to ingestion of saturated fat independent of obesity. A diet rich in simple sugars, as well as saturated fats increases the production of ROS by different mechanisms, including the effect on gut microbiota [13]. Lipid stimulated oxidative stress may be a key driver of insulin resistance and hyperandrogenism in PCOS. Excess adipose tissue is a contributor to the pro oxidant burden and an additional regulator of insulin action [14].Chronic exposure to androgens increases the oxidative stress in islet cells, inducing mitochondrial dysfunction [15, 16].

Superoxide is a ROS produced when NADPH is oxidized by membrane bound NADPH oxidase [17]. Dysregulation in ROS production from NADPH oxidase has been implicated in variety of disorders observed in women with PCOS like cardiovascular disorders, endothelial dysfunction, atherosclerosis and hypertension [18].

Peroxide induced oxidative stress activates nuclear factor k B (NF-kB), which in turn increases tumor necrosis factor (TNF)-alpha gene transcription [19].

Oxidative stress that occurs due to saturated fat ingestion is an intermediate step in stimulating TNF-alpha secretion from circulating leucocytes [14, 20]. The women with PCOS showed an increase in TNF-alpha synthesis [21].

Women with PCOS with normal or low levels of androgens measured by level of testosterone and free androgen index (FAI) were more susceptible to developing oxidative stress and inflammation by TNF-alpha [22].

An unhealthy diet is a key component of metabolic risk factors associated with PCOS pathophysiology along with hyperandrogenism, hyperinsulinemia and low grade chronic inflammation [23].

Eating disorders are also more prevalent in women with PCOS and hence all women with PCOS should be routinely screened for the same at the time of diagnosis [24].

13.3 Dietary Patterns and PCOS

For Finding a diet that can aid in prevention and treatment of PCOS one needs to understand the role of various diet patterns and their implication on PCOS.

13.3.1 Mediterranean Diet

The Mediterranean diet (MedDiet) is the healthiest dietary model due to its unique characteristics and has been included in international guidelines among recommended healthy dietary patterns.

It includes regular consumption of unsaturated fats, fiber, low glycemic index (low GI) carbohydrates, antioxidants and vitamins as well as appropriate amount of animal protein [24].

MedDiet reduces inflammation and oxidative stress markers and improves lipid profiles, insulin sensitivity, endothelial function as well as atherosclerotic and antithrombotic properties [25, 26].

Numerous studies over the years have shown that adopting a MedDiet can prevent against IR related diseases such as obesity, cardiovascular diseases, type 2 diabetes, non-alcoholic fatty liver (NAFLD), cognitive impairment, breast cancer and chronic kidney disease.

Considering there's a tight relationship between PCOS and obesity, chronic low grade inflammation and IR, MedDiet appears to be the one of the optimal non pharmacological strategies for the treatment of PCOS.

A recent study investigated the association between PCOS clinical severity, body composition and adherence to the MedDiet.

Women with PCOS consumed less extra virgin olive oil, legumes, fish, nuts compared to controls and consumed more simple carbohydrates, saturated fatty acids, PUFA's and n-6PUFA's; and consumed fewer complex carbohydrates, fiber, n-3PUFA's and monosaturated fatty acids than the control group.

There were positive associations between C-reactive protein, simple carbohydrates, saturated fatty acids, PUFA's and n-6PUFA's and negative correlations with consumption of protein, complex carbohydrates, fiber, n-3PUFA's and monosaturated fatty acids.

Among them n-3PUFA's supplementation is proven to improve insulin sensitivity and beneficial for metabolic management [27].

A negative correlation was reported between MedDiet and the clinical severity of PCOS; furthermore an unhealthy diet in women with PCOS contributed to more severe inflammation, IR, and hyperandrogenemia [26].

Another recent study found that patients consuming a predominantly pro inflammatory western diet and low consumption of fruits and vegetables led to chronic mucosal inflammation, impaired gut epithelial barrier and disturbances in gut microbiome while MedDiet has proven to fight inflammation by acting on the intestinal permeability, gut microbiome composition and inflammatory response.

It also improves the ovarian form (ovarian volume and follicle number per ovary [28]) by impacting obesity, IR, hyperandrogenism.

The beneficial effects of the MedDiet is due to the plant polyphenols obtained from the vegetables, fruits, legumes, grains, nuts, seeds and particularly red wine and extra virgin olive oil which has widely studied in the last several decades for its ability to reduce the metabolic syndrome [29].

Polyphenols reduce the inflammation and improves both the insulin sensitivity and compensatory hyperinsulinemia [30].

MedDiets are particularly rich in natural polyphenol called resveratrol, found in grapes, berries and wine which reduces androgen production and improves hyperandrogenism in PCOS [31].

13.3.2 Ketogenic Diet

The ketogenic or keto diet (KD) is a high fat and low carbohydrate diet that encourages giving up nearly all carbohydrates, consuming high levels of fat (exceeding 70% of calories consumed) and avoiding excess protein resulting in high production of ketones (acetoacetate and beta-hydroxybutyrate) and nutritional ketosis.

KD has been proposed as an effective diet for refractory epilepsy [32], other neurological disorders including Alzheimer's disease, Parkinsons disease and autism.

Research has shown its benefits in not only neurological but also gastrointestinal and endocrine diseases.

KD not only decreases the post prandial insulin secretion but it also reverses the IR by reducing weight, loss of fat mass, thereby helping to restore the function of insulin [33].

KD improves the menstrual cycle, reducing blood glucose and body weight, improving liver function, and treating fatty liver in obese women with PCOS and liver dysfunction.

A study showed that adhering to a 6 month low carbohydrate KD could help in reducing the androgen secretion, increase sex hormone binding globulin (SHBH) and improve insulin sensitivity, thereby renormalizing endocrine function, which in turn helps in the treatment of women with PCOS [34].

Paoli et al. [35]. studied 14 overweight women with PCOS who were on KD. It was observed that 12 weeks after dietary intervention, these women had significant reduction in anthropometric and body composition measurements. Reduction in body weight, body mass index (BMI), fat mass, visceral adipose tissue along with marked improvement in IR. All parameters related to PCOS also showed improvement including the LH/FSH ratio, levels of total LH, free testosterone, SHBH, DHEAS, estradiol and progesterone.

These results seem to point towards the beneficial effects of KD, suggesting this diet to be the optimal dietary intervention for patients of PCOS with advanced obesity and /or obesity accompanied by full blown metabolic syndrome.

13.3.3 Low Glycemic Diet (LGI)

Low GI diets are those that obtain most carbohydrate from low GI sources [36]. low GI foods are those foods having carbohydrates that are digested, absorbed and metabolized slowly that do not cause post prandial glycemia.

Post prandial glycemia increases the risk of lifestyle diseases and high glycemic diets may directly increase IR through their effect on glycemia, free fatty acids and counterregulatory hormone secretion [37] which goes on to suggest the importance of GI of contributing carbohydrate foods irrespective of the level of carbohydrate intake. Evidence shows that low GI diets helps in glycemic control, weight loss and lipid profile control [38].

A low GI diet compared to a normal GI diet improves ovulation cycles in patients with PCOS and anovulation [39].

A recent study showed low GI diets to be the optimal dietary choice for women with PCOS owing to its efficacy in improving the clinical manifestations of PCOS like IR, hyperandrogenism, menstrual irregularities as well as acne and hirsutism [40].

A preliminary report also showed that a low GI diet decreases endometrial thickness and increasing the number of menstrual cycles in women with PCOS that may reduce the risk of endometriosis [41].

13.3.4 Pulse Based High Fiber Diet

A pulse (e.g. Lentils, chickpeas, split beans, dry beans) based diet is high in fiber, low glycemic, low fat, contains high quality protein and complex carbohydrates, with significant amounts of vitamins, minerals such as iron, zinc, folate, calcium, magnesium and potassium [41].

Pulses alone or along with a low GI or high fiber diets improve the glycemic control in humans. It has been used to maintain insulin sensitivity and reduce the IR [42]. consuming pulses have shown to reduce the risk of metabolic disease in PCOS patients.

Phytochemicals like saponins and tannins are known for its anti-cancer effects that may reduce the endometrial cancer risk in women with PCOS [43].

13.4 Conclusion

Dietary interventions may improve reproductive and metabolic function.

Weight loss showed improvement in presentation of PCOS regardless of type and composition of diet in the majority of dietary studies.

Women with PCOS when gain weight resulting in obesity can aggravate the phenotype of infertility, anovulation, metabolic alterations and menstrual abnormalities [44].

Adipose tissue is an extraglandular source of androgens especially abdominal obesity and can worsen hyperandrogenism [35].

In conclusion, all women with PCOS should incorporate healthy lifestyle, healthy eating and regular physical activity to improve overall health that can contribute in optimizing hormonal outcomes, general health and quality of life.

However, more research and studies are required to support long term efficacy, safety and health benefits of these diets in PCOS.

References

1. Fauser BCJM, Tarlatzis BC, Rebar RW, Legro RS, Balen AH, Lobo R, Carmina E, Chang J, Yildiz BO, Laven JSE, et al. Consensus on women's health aspects of polycystic ovary syndrome (PCOS): The Amsterdam ESHRE/ASRM-sponsored 3rd PCOS Consensus Workshop Group. Fertil Steril. 2012;97:28–38.e25. https://doi.org/10.1016/j.fertnstert.2011.09.024.
2. Azziz R. Polycystic ovary syndrome. Obstet Gynecol. 2018;132(2):321–36. https://doi.org/10.1097/AOG.0000000000002698.
3. Del Pup L, Cagnacci A. IMPROVE lifestyle in polycystic ovary syndrome: a systematic strategy. Gynecol Endocrinol. 2021;37:1–4. https://doi.org/10.1080/09513590.2021.1871892.
4. Szczuko M, Skowronek M, Zapałowska-Chwyć M, Starczewski A. Quantitative assessment of nutrition in patients with polycystic ovary syndrome (PCOS). Rocz Panstw Zakl Hig. 2016;67:419–26.
5. Makki K, Froguel P, Wolowczuk I. Adipose tissue in obesity-related inflammation and insulin resistance: cells, cytokines, and chemokines. ISRN Inflamm. 2013;2013:139239. https://doi.org/10.1155/2013/139239.
6. Szczuko M, Sankowska P, Zapałowska-Chwyć M, Wysokiński P. Studies on the quality nutrition in women with polycystic ovary syndrome (PCOS). Rocz Panstw Zakl Hig. 2017;68(1):61–7.

7. Tremellen K, Pearce K. Dysbiosis of gut microbiota (DOGMA): a novel theory for the development of polycystic ovarian syndrome. Med Hypotheses. 2012;79(1):104–12. https://doi.org/10.1016/j.mehy.2012.04.016.
8. Jiao N, Baker SS, Nugent CA, Tsompana M, Cai L, Wang Y, Buck MJ, Genco RJ, Baker RD, Zhu R, et al. Gut microbiome may contribute to insulin resistance and systemic inflammation in obese rodents: a meta-analysis. Physiol Genomics. 2018;50:244–54. https://doi.org/10.1152/physiolgenomics.00114.2017.
9. Zhang Z, Bai L, Guan M, Zhou X, Liang X, Lv Y, Yi H, Zhou H, Liu T, Gong P, et al. Potential probiotics Lactobacillus casei K11 combined with plant extracts reduce markers of type 2 diabetes mellitus in mice. J Appl Microbiol. 2021;131:1970. https://doi.org/10.1111/jam.15061.
10. Bamberger C, Rossmeier A, Lechner K, Wu L, Waldmann E, Fischer S, Stark RG, Altenhofer J, Henze K, Parhofer KG. A Walnut-enriched diet affects gut microbiome in healthy caucasian subjects: a randomized, controlled trial. Nutrients. 2018;10:244. https://doi.org/10.3390/nu10020244.
11. Zhang Z, Bai L, Guan M, Zhou X, Liang X, Lv Y, Yi H, Zhou H, Liu T, Gong P, et al. Potential probiotics Lactobacillus casei K11 combined with plant extracts reduce markers of type 2 diabetes mellitus in mice. J Appl Microbiol. 2021;131:1970.
12. den Besten G, van Eunen K, Groen AK, Venema K, Reijngoud D-J, Bakker BM. The role of short-chain fatty acids in the interplay between diet, gut microbiota, and host energy metabolism. J Lipid Res. 2013;54:2325–40. https://doi.org/10.1194/jlr.R036012.
13. Fajstova A, Galanova N, Coufal S, Malkova J, Kostovcik M, Cermakova M, Pelantova H, Kuzma M, Sediva B, Hudcovic T, et al. Diet rich in simple sugars promotes pro-inflammatory response via gut microbiota alteration and TLR4 signaling. Cells. 2020;9:2701. https://doi.org/10.3390/cells9122701.
14. González F, Considine RV, Abdelhadi OA, Acton AJ. Oxidative stress in response to saturated fat ingestion is linked to insulin resistance and hyperandrogenism in polycystic ovary syndrome. J Clin Endocrinol Metab. 2019;104:5360–71. https://doi.org/10.1210/jc.2019-00987.
15. Wang H, Wang X, Zhu Y, Chen F, Sun Y, Han X. Increased androgen levels in rats impair glucose-stimulated insulin secretion through disruption of pancreatic beta cell mitochondrial function. J Steroid Biochem Mol Biol. 2015;154:254–66. https://doi.org/10.1016/j.jsbmb.2015.09.003.
16. Liu S, Navarro G, Mauvais-Jarvis F. Androgen excess produces systemic oxidative stress and predisposes to beta-cell failure in female mice. PLoS One. 2010;5:e11302. https://doi.org/10.1371/journal.pone.0011302.
17. Jiang F, Zhang Y, Dusting GJ. NADPH oxidase-mediated redox signaling: roles in cellular stress response, stress tolerance, and tissue repair. Pharm Rev. 2011;63:218–42. https://doi.org/10.1124/pr.110.002980.
18. Bedard K, Krause K-H. The NOX family of ROS-generating NADPH oxidases: physiology and pathophysiology. Physiol Rev. 2007;87:245–313. https://doi.org/10.1152/physrev.00044.2005.
19. Evans JL, Goldfine ID, Maddux BA, Grodsky GM. Oxidative stress and stress-activated signaling pathways: a unifying hypothesis of type 2 diabetes. Endocr Rev. 2002;23:599–622. https://doi.org/10.1210/er.2001-0039.
20. González F, Considine RV, Abdelhadi OA, Acton AJ. Saturated fat ingestion promotes lipopolysaccharide-mediated inflammation and insulin resistance in polycystic ovary syndrome. J Clin Endocrinol Metab. 2018;104:934–46. https://doi.org/10.1210/jc.2018-01143.
21. Ma L, Cao Y, Ma Y, Zhai J. Association between hyperandrogenism and adverse pregnancy outcomes in patients with different polycystic ovary syndrome phenotypes undergoing in vitro fertilization/intracytoplasmic sperm injection: a systematic review and meta-analysis. Gynecol Endocrinol. 2021;37:1–8. https://doi.org/10.1080/09513590.2021.1897096.
22. Szczuko M, Zapałowska-Chwyć M, Maciejewska D, Drozd A, Starczewski A, Stachowska E. High glycemic index diet in PCOS patients. The analysis of IGF I and TNF-α pathways in metabolic disorders. Med Hypotheses. 2016;96:42–7. https://doi.org/10.1016/j.mehy.2016.09.016.

23. Barrea L, Marzullo P, Muscogiuri G, Di Somma C, Scacchi M, Orio F. Source and amount of carbohydrate in the diet and inflammation in women with polycystic ovary syndrome. Nutr Res Rev. 2018;31(2):291–301. https://doi.org/10.1017/S0954422418000136.
24. Dokras A, Stener-Victorin E, Yildiz BO, Li R, Ottey S, Shah D. Androgen excess- polycystic ovary syndrome society: position statement on depression, anxiety, quality of life, and eating disorders in polycystic ovary syndrome. Fertil Steril. 2018;109(5):888–99. https://doi.org/10.1016/j.fertnstert.2018.01.038.
25. Barrea L, Arnone A, Annunziata G, Muscogiuri G, Laudision D, Salzano C. Adherence to the mediterranean diet, dietary patterns and body composition in women with polycystic ovary syndrome (PCOS). Nutrients. 2019;11(10):1. https://doi.org/10.3390/nu11102278.
26. Martinez-Gonzalez MA, Salas-Salvado J, Estruch R, Corella D, Fito M, Ros E. Benefits of the mediterranean diet: insights from the PREDIMED Study. Prog Cardiovasc Dis. 2015;58(1):50–60.
27. Ditano-Vazquez P, Torres-Pena JD, Galeano-Valle F, Perez-Caballero AI, Demelo-Rodriguez P, Lopez-Miranda J. The fluid aspect of the mediterranean diet in the prevention and management of cardiovascular disease and diabetes: the role of polyphenol content in moderate consumption of wine and olive oil. Nutrients. 2019;11(11):2833.
28. Frias-Toral E, Garcia-Velasquez E, de Los Angeles Carignano M, Rodriguez-Veintimilla D, Alvarado-AguileraI, Bautista-Litardo N. Polycystic ovary syndrome and obesity: clinical aspects and nutritional management. Minerva Endocrinol. 2021;47:215.
29. Kazemi M, Jarrett BY, Vanden Brink H, Lin AW, Hoeger KM, Spandorfer SD. Obesity, insulin resistance, and hyperandrogenism mediate the link between poor diet quality and ovarian dysmorphology in reproductive-aged women. Nutrients. 2020;12(7):1953. https://doi.org/10.3390/nu12071953.
30. Leri M, Scuto M, Ontario ML, Calabrese V, Calabrese EJ, Bucciantini M. Healthy effects of plant polyphenols: molecular mechanisms. Int J Mol Sci. 2020;21(4):1250. https://doi.org/10.3390/ijms21041250.
31. Piroddi M, Albini A, Fabiani R, Giovannelli L, Luceri C, Natella F. Nutrigenomics of extra-virgin olive oil: a review. Biofactors. 2017;43(1):17–41. https://doi.org/10.1002/biof.1318.
32. Mirabelli M, Chiefari E, Arcidiacono B, Corigliano DM, Brunetti FS, Maggisano V. Mediterranean diet nutrients to turn the tide against insulin resistance and related diseases. Nutrients. 2020;12(4):1066. https://doi.org/10.3390/nu12041066.
33. Kuchkuntla AR, Shah M, Velapati S, Gershuni VM, Rajjo T, Nanda S. Ketogenic diet: an endocrinologist perspective. Curr Nutr Rep. 2019;8(4):402–10. https://doi.org/10.1007/s13668-019-00297-x.
34. Mavropoulos JC, Yancy WS, Hepburn J, Westman EC. The effects of a low-carbohydrate, ketogenic diet on the polycystic ovary syndrome: a pilot study. Nutr Metab. 2005;2:35. https://doi.org/10.1186/1743-7075-2-35.
35. Paoli A, Mancin L, Giacona MC, Bianco A, Caprio M. Effects of a ketogenic diet in overweight women with polycystic ovary syndrome. J Transl Med. 2020;18(1):104. https://doi.org/10.1186/s12967-020-02277-0.
36. Augustin LS, Kendall CW, Jenkins DJ, Willett WC, Astrup A, Barclay AW. Glycemic index, glycemic load and glycemic response: an international scientific consensus summit from the international carbohydrate quality consortium (ICQC). Nutr Metab Cardiovasc Dis. 2015;25(9):795–815. https://doi.org/10.1016/j.numecd.2015.05.005.
37. Barclay AW, Petocz P, McMillan-Price J, Flood VM, Prvan T, Mitchell P. Glycemic index, glycemic load, and chronic disease risk: a meta-analysis of observational studies. Am J Clin Nutr. 2008;87(3):627–37. https://doi.org/10.1093/ajcn/87.3.627.
38. Zafar MI, Mills KE, Zheng J, Regmi A, Hu SQ, Gou L. Low-glycemic index diets as an intervention for diabetes: a systematic review and meta-analysis. Am J Clin Nutr. 2019;110(4):891–902. https://doi.org/10.1093/ajcn/nqz149.
39. Sordia-Hernandez LH, Ancer Rodriguez P, Saldivar Rodriguez D, Trejo Guzman S, Servin Zenteno ES, Guerrero Gonzalez G. Effect of a low glycemic diet in patients with polycystic

ovary syndrome and anovulation—a randomized controlled trial. Clin Exp Obstet Gynecol. 2016;43(4):555–9.

40. Atiomo W, Read A, Golding M, Silcocks P, Sarkar RN. Local recruitment experience in a study comparing the effectiveness of a low glycaemic index diet with a low calorie healthy eating approach at achieving weight loss and reducing the risk of endometrial cancer in women with polycystic ovary syndrome (PCOS). Contemp Clin Trials. 2009;30(5):451–6. https://doi.org/10.1016/j.cct.2009.05.001.
41. Mudryj AN, Yu N, Aukema HM. Nutritional and health benefits of pulses. Appl Physiol Nutr Metab. 2014;39(11):1197–204. https://doi.org/10.1139/apnm-2013-0557.
42. Sievenpiper JL, Kendall CW, Esfahani A, Wong JM, Carleton AJ, Jiang HY. Effect of non-oil-seed pulses on glycaemic control: a systematic review and meta-analysis of randomised controlled experimental trials in people with and without diabetes. Diabetologia. 2009;52(8):1479–95. https://doi.org/10.1007/s00125-009-1395-7.
43. Charalampakis V, Tahrani AA, Helmy A, Gupta JK, Singhal R. Polycystic ovary syndrome and endometrial hyperplasia: an overview of the role of bariatric surgery in female fertility. Eur J Obstet Gynecol Reprod Biol. 2016;207:220–6. https://doi.org/10.1016/j.ejogrb.2016.10.001.
44. Conway G, Dewailly D, Diamanti-Kandarakis E, Escobar-Morreale HF, Franks S, Gambineri A. The polycystic ovary syndrome: a position statement from the European society of endocrinology. Eur J Endocrinol. 2014;171(4):P1–29. https://doi.org/10.1530/EJE-14-0253.

Chapter 14
Urticaria and Hormones

Tania Yadav

14.1 Introduction

Urticaria is a common dermatological condition characterized by the development of red, itchy, raised skin lesions, which can be triggered by a wide range of factors including infections, allergens, drugs, and physical stimuli. These eruptions last for a few hours but not exceeding 48 h. The term angioneurotic oedema denotes larger swellings of the deep dermal, sub-cutaneous and sub mucosal tissues Hormones are known to play a role in the pathogenesis of urticaria, as they can modulate the immune response and increase the susceptibility of the skin to environmental triggers. In this chapter, we will discuss the relationship between urticaria and hormones, with a particular focus on estrogen, progesterone, and thyroid hormones [1–3].

14.2 Thyroid and Urticaria

The thyroid hormone has been implicated in the pathogenesis of urticaria, with a higher prevalence of thyroid abnormalities found in patients with chronic urticaria.

T. Yadav (✉)
Dermcos Clinic & Medanta Hospital, Gurgaon, Haryana, India

R. Singh, N. Sharma (eds.), *A Guide to Hormonal Dermatology*,
https://doi.org/10.1007/978-981-99-7715-4_14

14.2.1 Pathogenesis

The exact pathogenesis of thyroid hormone-associated urticaria remains unclear. However, it is thought that thyroid hormones affect the immune system by altering the levels of cytokines, T-lymphocyte subsets, and immunoglobulin synthesis. Thyroid hormones also play a role in mast cell activation, which is a key player in the development of urticaria [3].

14.2.2 Predisposing Factors

Several factors increase the risk of developing urticaria in patients with thyroid abnormalities, including autoimmune thyroid disease, female sex, and older age. Additionally, patients with chronic urticaria are more likely to have thyroid abnormalities, with a prevalence ranging from 10 to 40% depending on the study.

14.2.3 Urticaria and Thyroid Abnormality Associations

A significant association has been reported between thyroid abnormalities and chronic urticaria. A study by Kaplan et al. found that 22% of patients with chronic urticaria had elevated thyroid antibodies compared to 6% of control subjects ($p < 0.01$) (Kaplan et al., 1987). In a meta-analysis by Ferrer et al., thyroid abnormalities were found in 27% of patients with chronic urticaria compared to 9% of control subjects ($p < 0.001$) (Ferrer et al. 2002) [4, 5].

14.2.4 Clinical Features

Patients with thyroid hormone-associated urticaria present with typical urticarial lesions, including raised, erythematous, and pruritic wheals that may be accompanied by angioedema. However, these patients may also have symptoms of thyroid dysfunction, including weight changes, fatigue, hair loss, and menstrual irregularities.

14.2.5 Diagnosis

The diagnosis of thyroid hormone-associated urticaria requires a thorough medical history, physical examination, and laboratory investigations. Thyroid function tests, including serum levels of thyroid-stimulating hormone (TSH), free thyroxine (T4), and triiodothyronine (T3), should be performed. Elevated levels of thyroid antibodies, including anti-thyroglobulin (TgAb) and anti-thyroid peroxidase (TPOAb), may also be present in these patients [6].

14.2.6 Treatment

The treatment of thyroid hormone-associated urticaria depends on the underlying thyroid abnormality. In patients with hypothyroidism, replacement therapy with levothyroxine may be effective in controlling both urticaria and thyroid dysfunction. In patients with hyperthyroidism, treatment may involve anti-thyroid medications or radioactive iodine therapy. Antihistamines are also commonly used to control symptoms of urticaria in these patients [7, 8].

14.3 Estrogen and Urticaria

Estrogen, a hormone responsible for the development and maintenance of female sexual characteristics, has been implicated in the pathogenesis of urticaria.

14.3.1 Pathogenesis

The exact pathogenesis of urticaria associated with estrogen is not well understood. However, it is believed that estrogen may trigger urticaria through its effects on mast cells, which are responsible for the release of histamine, cytokines, and other mediators of inflammation.

Estrogen has been shown to increase the expression of mast cell tryptase, a protease that activates the complement system and cleaves other mediators of inflammation. Additionally, estrogen may increase the sensitivity of mast cells to stimuli such as allergens or physical stimuli, leading to the release of inflammatory mediators [9].

14.3.2 Clinical Features

Urticaria associated with estrogen can occur at any age, but it is most common in women during periods of hormonal fluctuations, such as pregnancy, menstrual cycle, and menopause. The lesions of estrogen-induced urticaria are typically pruritic, erythematous wheals that may coalesce to form larger plaques. The rash is usually located on the trunk, but can also occur on the extremities, face, and scalp.

14.3.3 Diagnosis

The diagnosis of urticaria associated with estrogen is primarily based on the patient's history and clinical examination. A thorough medical history, including menstrual cycle status, pregnancy history, and contraceptive use, should be obtained. Physical examination should include a careful inspection of the skin, as well as an assessment of the patient's general health.

Additional diagnostic tests may be ordered, including skin prick testing, radioallergosorbent testing (RAST), and laboratory tests to measure estrogen levels. However, these tests are not always necessary and are generally only performed when other causes of urticaria have been ruled out [10].

14.3.4 Treatment

The treatment of urticaria associated with estrogen involves both the identification and avoidance of triggering factors and the use of pharmacotherapy. Treatment options include antihistamines, corticosteroids, and immune modulators.

Antihistamines are the first-line treatment for urticaria and work by blocking the effects of histamine. Second-generation antihistamines, such as cetirizine and fexofenadine, are preferred due to their effectiveness and reduced side effects compared to first-generation antihistamines such as diphenhydramine.

Corticosteroids, such as prednisone, may be used in severe cases or in combination with antihistamines. However, they are generally reserved for short-term use due to the risk of side effects such as osteoporosis and adrenal suppression.

Immune modulators, such as omalizumab, are effective in treating chronic urticaria and may be considered in refractory cases. Omalizumab is a monoclonal antibody that binds to IgE, preventing its binding to mast cells and subsequent activation [11].

14.4 Progesterone and Urticaria

In recent years, the role of hormones, particularly progesterone, in the development of urticaria has been studied extensively.

14.4.1 Pathogenesis

Progesterone is a hormone that is produced by the ovaries during the menstrual cycle and plays a vital role in preparing the uterus for pregnancy. It has also been found to have a significant impact on the immune system, particularly in women.

Progesterone has been shown to stimulate the production of certain cytokines and chemokines, which can trigger an inflammatory response and cause urticaria. Furthermore, it has been proposed that progesterone may also activate mast cells, which are key players in the pathogenesis of urticaria [4, 12, 13].

14.4.2 Clinical Features

The clinical features of progesterone-induced urticaria can vary depending on the individual. The most common symptoms include the sudden onset of itchy, red wheals on the skin, which may be accompanied by swelling and pain. The rash may be localized or spread across the body and can last for several days. In some cases, symptoms may worsen during the menstrual cycle when progesterone levels are at their highest [14].

14.4.3 Diagnosis

The diagnosis of progesterone-induced urticaria can be challenging as the symptoms are often nonspecific and can mimic other conditions. However, a thorough medical history and physical examination can help identify potential triggers, such as hormonal fluctuations. In some cases, skin testing or blood tests may be necessary to confirm the diagnosis.

14.4.4 Clinical Implications

Progesterone-induced urticaria can have significant clinical implications, particularly in women of childbearing age. The condition can cause significant discomfort and may interfere with daily activities. Additionally, it may indicate an underlying hormonal imbalance that requires further investigation and treatment [12, 15].

14.4.5 Associations

Progesterone-induced urticaria has been associated with various conditions, including autoimmune disorders such as systemic lupus erythematosus, and rheumatoid arthritis. It has also been reported in women who are pregnant or taking hormonal contraceptives.

14.4.6 *Treatment*

The treatment of progesterone-induced urticaria depends on the severity of symptoms and the underlying cause. Antihistamines are the first-line treatment for mild cases and can help relieve itching and reduce the size and number of wheals. In more severe cases, oral corticosteroids or immunosuppressive agents may be necessary. Hormonal therapy, such as the use of progesterone antagonists, has also been shown to be effective in some cases [11, 16, 17].

14.5 Metabolic Syndrome and Urticaria

Metabolic syndrome is a cluster of medical conditions including obesity, insulin resistance, dyslipidemia, and hypertension that are associated with increased risk of cardiovascular diseases, type 2 diabetes, and other chronic diseases. Recent studies suggest that metabolic syndrome may also play a role in the pathogenesis of urticaria. Urticaria, commonly known as hives, is a skin disorder characterized by itchy, raised, red welts that occur in response to various stimuli. This chapter aims to explore the link between metabolic syndromes and urticaria, including pathogenesis, predisposing factors, clinical features, clinical implications, associations, diagnosis, and treatment [18].

14.5.1 *Pathogenesis*

The pathogenesis of urticaria involves the release of histamine and other proinflammatory mediators from mast cells in response to various stimuli, including allergens, infections, and physical factors. The exact mechanisms linking metabolic syndrome and urticaria are not fully understood. However, it is hypothesized that insulin resistance and chronic inflammation associated with metabolic syndrome may trigger mast cell activation and histamine release, leading to the development of urticaria.

14.5.2 *Predisposing Factors*

Obesity is a well-established risk factor for metabolic syndrome, and recent studies suggest that it may also increase the risk of urticaria. Other factors associated with both metabolic syndrome and urticaria include sedentary lifestyle, unhealthy diet, and stress. Genetic factors may also play a role in the development of both conditions [19].

14.5.3 Clinical Features

Urticaria typically presents as itchy, raised, red welts on the skin that may appear and disappear quickly. The lesions may vary in size and shape and may be distributed all over the body. In some cases, urticaria may be accompanied by angioedema, which involves swelling of the deeper layers of the skin and mucous membranes. Patients with metabolic syndrome and urticaria may also exhibit other clinical features of metabolic syndrome, including obesity, insulin resistance, dyslipidemia, and hypertension [20].

14.5.4 Clinical Implications

The presence of urticaria in patients with metabolic syndrome may indicate an increased risk of cardiovascular diseases and other chronic conditions associated with metabolic syndrome. Patients with both conditions may require more aggressive management of their metabolic syndrome to reduce the risk of these complications [21, 22].

14.5.5 Associations

Several studies have investigated the association between metabolic syndrome and urticaria. A study published in the Journal of Allergy and Clinical Immunology found that patients with chronic urticaria were more likely to have metabolic syndrome than those without urticaria. Another study published in the Journal of Dermatology found that patients with chronic spontaneous urticaria had higher levels of insulin resistance compared to healthy controls. These findings suggest that there may be a link between metabolic syndrome and urticarial [23].

14.5.6 Diagnosis

Diagnosis of urticaria is typically based on clinical features, including the appearance of itchy, raised, red wheals on the skin. In some cases, laboratory tests may be ordered to identify underlying causes of urticaria, including allergens, infections, or autoimmune disorders. Diagnosis of metabolic syndrome is based on the presence of at least three of the following conditions: obesity, insulin resistance, dyslipidemia, and hypertension [21, 22, 24, 25].

14.5.7 *Treatment*

Treatment of urticaria typically involves the use of antihistamines to block the effects of histamine on the skin. In patients with metabolic syndrome and urticaria, management of metabolic syndrome may also be necessary to reduce the risk of cardiovascular diseases and other complications. Lifestyle modifications, including weight loss, healthy diet, and regular exercise, may be effective in improving metabolic syndrome and reducing the severity of urticaria. In some cases, medications to lower blood pressure, control blood sugar, or lower cholesterol levels may also be necessary [26].

14.6 Conclusion

In conclusion, hormones have been found to play a significant role in the development of urticaria. The complex interplay between various hormones and immune system components is still being explored by medical researchers.

Presently, various medications and treatments are available for urticaria, including antihistamines, corticosteroids, and immunomodulatory drugs. However, these treatments may not be effective for all patients, and more research is needed to develop new therapies that target the underlying hormonal imbalances.

The medical world is actively working to uncover more insights into the complex relationship between hormones and urticaria. Recent studies have highlighted the potential therapeutic benefits of targeting specific hormones, such as thyrotropin-releasing hormone, in the treatment of urticaria.

Overall, while there is still much to be learned about the role of hormones in urticaria, ongoing research offers hope for improved treatment options and better outcomes for patients.

References

1. Prasad PS. Urticaria. Indian J Dermatol Venereol Leprol. 2001;67:11–20.
2. Kasperska-Zajac A, Brzoza Z, Rogala B. Sex hormones and urticaria. J Dermatol Sci. 2008;52(2):79–86.
3. Gonzalez-Diaz SN, Sanchez-Borges M, Rangel-Gonzalez DM, Guzman-Avilan RI, Canseco-Villarreal JI, Arias-Cruz A. Chronic urticaria and thyroid pathology. World Allergy Organ J. 2020;13(3):100101.
4. Kaplan AP, Greaves MW. Pathogenesis of chronic urticaria. Clin Exp Allergy. 1987;17(Suppl 1):19–22.
5. Ferrer M, Bartra J, Giménez-Arnau A, et al. Management of urticaria: not too complicated, not too simple. Clin Exp Allergy. 2015;45(2):301–12.
6. Grattan CEH, Wallington TB, Warin RP, et al. A Serological and Clinical Evaluation of Chronic Urticaria. Br J Dermatol. 1986;114(5):583–90.

7. Gomaa NH, Elgendy D, Fawzy MM, et al. Study of thyroid abnormalities in patients with chronic urticaria: a hospital-based study in Upper Egypt. Egypt J Dermatol Venerol. 2019;39(2):13–9.
8. Pajunk R, Altrichter S, Bieber T, et al. Classification and management of chronic urticaria patients with thyroid autoantibodies: a systematic review and consensus-based statement. J Eur Acad Dermatol Venereol. 2022;36(1):6–20.
9. Kasperska-Zając A, Grzanka A. Estrogen and chronic urticaria. Postepy Dermatol Alergol. 2015;32(3):178–82.
10. Tauscher AE, Schaefer P. Urticaria and angioedema. Am Fam Physician. 2007;76(10): 1517–22.
11. Zuberbier T, Aberer W, Asero R, et al. The EAACI/GA²LEN/EDF/WAO guideline for the definition, classification, diagnosis and management of urticaria. Allergy. 2018;73(7):1393–414.
12. Kim M, Lee KH. Urticaria induced by female hormones: a review. J Dermatol Sci. 2018;91(1):3–9.
13. Grattan CE, Wallington TB. Urticaria and angioedema. In: Davidson's principles and practice of medicine, vol. 69. Amsterdam: Elsevier; 2004. p. 1317–20.
14. Hart R. Autoimmune progesterone dermatitis. Arch Dermatol. 1977;113(4):426–30.
15. Mahlab G, Mimouni M, Kidron D. Progesterone-induced dermatitis. J Am Acad Dermatol. 1990;22(2):330–2.
16. Krause K, Grattan CE, Bindslev-Jensen C. Progesterone and urticaria. Skin Ther Lett. 2015;20(4):5–7.
17. Zanotti R, Lombardi C, Girolomoni G, Senna G. Chronic urticaria: new insights from recent guidelines and the role of current and future therapies. J Asthma Aller. 2013;6:65–77.
18. Mendelson L, Falanga V. Urticaria and angioedema. In: Wolff K, Goldsmith LA, Katz SI, et al., editors. Fitzpatrick's Dermatology in General Medicine. 7th ed. New York: McGraw-Hill; 2008. p. 487–502.
19. Grundy SM, Brewer HB Jr, Cleeman JI, Smith SC Jr, Lenfant C. Definition of metabolic syndrome: report of the National Heart, Lung, and Blood Institute/American Heart Association conference on scientific issues related to definition. Circulation. 2004;109(3):433–8.
20. Sánchez J, Amaya E, Acevedo A, et al. Urticaria and urticaria-like dermatoses: an update. Actas Dermosifiliogr. 2015;106(2):88–98.
21. Maurer M, Weller K, Bindslev-Jensen C, et al. Unmet clinical needs in chronic spontaneous urticaria. A GA²LEN task force report. Allergy. 2011;66(3):317–30.
22. Ye YM, Park HS. Recent advances in understanding and managing chronic urticaria. F1000Res. 2019;8:F1000 Faculty Rev-1239.
23. Rabelo-Filardi R, Ferreira-Machado AB, Kac G. Association between urticaria and metabolic syndrome: a systematic review. Allergy Asthma Proc. 2017;38(4):260–6.
24. Mlynek A, Magerl M, Hanna M, et al. The German version of the Chronic Urticaria Quality of Life Questionnaire: factor analysis, validation, and initial clinical findings. Allergy. 2009;64(6):927–36.
25. Ertugrul DT, Karadag AS, Tutal E, Akin KO. Insulin resistance in patients with chronic spontaneous urticaria: a case-control study. Am J Clin Dermatol. 2014;15(3):257–61.
26. Grattan CE, Humphreys F. Guidelines for evaluation and management of urticaria in adults and children. Br J Dermatol. 2007;157(6):1116–23.

MIX
Papier aus verantwortungsvollen Quellen
Paper from responsible sources
FSC® C105338

If you have any concerns about our products,
you can contact us on
ProductSafety@springernature.com

In case Publisher is established outside the EU,
the EU authorized representative is:
Springer Nature Customer Service Center GmbH
Europaplatz 3, 69115 Heidelberg, Germany

Printed by Libri Plureos GmbH
in Hamburg, Germany

7. Gomaa NH, Elgendy D, Fawzy MM, et al. Study of thyroid abnormalities in patients with chronic urticaria: a hospital-based study in Upper Egypt. Egypt J Dermatol Venerol. 2019;39(2):13–9.
8. Pajunk R, Altrichter S, Bieber T, et al. Classification and management of chronic urticaria patients with thyroid autoantibodies: a systematic review and consensus-based statement. J Eur Acad Dermatol Venereol. 2022;36(1):6–20.
9. Kasperska-Zając A, Grzanka A. Estrogen and chronic urticaria. Postepy Dermatol Alergol. 2015;32(3):178–82.
10. Tauscher AE, Schaefer P. Urticaria and angioedema. Am Fam Physician. 2007;76(10): 1517–22.
11. Zuberbier T, Aberer W, Asero R, et al. The EAACI/GA^{2}LEN/EDF/WAO guideline for the definition, classification, diagnosis and management of urticaria. Allergy. 2018;73(7):1393–414.
12. Kim M, Lee KH. Urticaria induced by female hormones: a review. J Dermatol Sci. 2018;91(1):3–9.
13. Grattan CE, Wallington TB. Urticaria and angioedema. In: Davidson's principles and practice of medicine, vol. 69. Amsterdam: Elsevier; 2004. p. 1317–20.
14. Hart R. Autoimmune progesterone dermatitis. Arch Dermatol. 1977;113(4):426–30.
15. Mahlab G, Mimouni M, Kidron D. Progesterone-induced dermatitis. J Am Acad Dermatol. 1990;22(2):330–2.
16. Krause K, Grattan CE, Bindslev-Jensen C. Progesterone and urticaria. Skin Ther Lett. 2015;20(4):5–7.
17. Zanotti R, Lombardi C, Girolomoni G, Senna G. Chronic urticaria: new insights from recent guidelines and the role of current and future therapies. J Asthma Aller. 2013;6:65–77.
18. Mendelson L, Falanga V. Urticaria and angioedema. In: Wolff K, Goldsmith LA, Katz SI, et al., editors. Fitzpatrick's Dermatology in General Medicine. 7th ed. New York: McGraw-Hill; 2008. p. 487–502.
19. Grundy SM, Brewer HB Jr, Cleeman JI, Smith SC Jr, Lenfant C. Definition of metabolic syndrome: report of the National Heart, Lung, and Blood Institute/American Heart Association conference on scientific issues related to definition. Circulation. 2004;109(3):433–8.
20. Sánchez J, Amaya E, Acevedo A, et al. Urticaria and urticaria-like dermatoses: an update. Actas Dermosifiliogr. 2015;106(2):88–98.
21. Maurer M, Weller K, Bindslev-Jensen C, et al. Unmet clinical needs in chronic spontaneous urticaria. A GA^{2}LEN task force report. Allergy. 2011;66(3):317–30.
22. Ye YM, Park HS. Recent advances in understanding and managing chronic urticaria. F1000Res. 2019;8:F1000 Faculty Rev-1239.
23. Rabelo-Filardi R, Ferreira-Machado AB, Kac G. Association between urticaria and metabolic syndrome: a systematic review. Allergy Asthma Proc. 2017;38(4):260–6.
24. Mlynek A, Magerl M, Hanna M, et al. The German version of the Chronic Urticaria Quality of Life Questionnaire: factor analysis, validation, and initial clinical findings. Allergy. 2009;64(6):927–36.
25. Ertugrul DT, Karadag AS, Tutal E, Akin KO. Insulin resistance in patients with chronic spontaneous urticaria: a case-control study. Am J Clin Dermatol. 2014;15(3):257–61.
26. Grattan CE, Humphreys F. Guidelines for evaluation and management of urticaria in adults and children. Br J Dermatol. 2007;157(6):1116–23.

MIX
Papier aus verantwortungsvollen Quellen
Paper from responsible sources
FSC® C105338

If you have any concerns about our products,
you can contact us on
ProductSafety@springernature.com

In case Publisher is established outside the EU,
the EU authorized representative is:
Springer Nature Customer Service Center GmbH
Europaplatz 3, 69115 Heidelberg, Germany

Printed by Libri Plureos GmbH
in Hamburg, Germany